Just What the Doctor Ordered

A COMPLETE GUIDE TO DRUGS AND MEDICATIONS FOR YOUR DOG

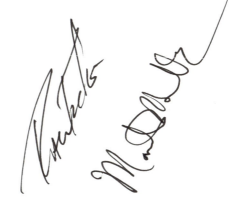

Race Foster, D.V.M.

Marty Smith, D.V.M.

HOWELL
BOOK
HOUSE

New York

Howell Book House
A Simon and Schuster Macmillan Company
1633 Broadway
New York, NY 10019

Library of Congress Cataloging-in-Publication Data

Foster, Race.

Just what the doctor ordered : a complete guide to drugs and medications for your dog/Race Foster, Marty Smith.

     p. cm.

  Includes bibliographical references.

  ISBN 0-87605-787-3

  1. Dogs—Diseases—Chemotherapy. 2. Veterinary drugs. I. Smith, Marty. II. Title.

SF991.F575 1996

636.7'08951—dc20   96-22099

                                                   CIP

Manufactured in the United States of America

10 9 8 7 6 5 4 3 2 1

Design by Kris Tobiassen

Contents

Acknowledgments

It is appropriate to thank all of the responsible pet owners who make the Doctors Foster and Smith company a reality.

As veterinarians we have dedicated our lives to serving you; and because of that, the employees of Doctors Foster and Smith have trained to become educated in the care of animals. We appreciate the fact that they take pride in being a part of our company. In fact, they *are* the company.

Lastly, certain employees have worked long and hard on this particular project. A special thanks to SueEllen Hopp, Candi Besaw, Tanya Frisque, Cindy Alsteen, and Pati Dinda in providing expertise in assembling this book. Marcy Zingler of Howell Book House provided much professional support when it was needed.

This book is dedicated with love to our wives Kathy and Lynne and our children: Amanda, Megan, Katrina, Jessica, Johannah, Trenton, Tristan, Katie, and Keaton.

They are the ones who patiently allowed us to spend our evenings with books and computers while we worked on this endeavor.

Introduction

When a child is taken to a pediatrician or a pet visits a veterinarian, a certain protocol is followed. A detailed history of the patient and relevant ailments is taken. Secondly, the patient is subjected to a physical examination to search for clues about the ailment. Thirdly, sophisticated laboratory tests may be performed, including radiographs, EKGs and blood chemistries. Hopefully these procedures will yield a diagnosis so the appropriate therapy can be decided, if needed. Treatment may include nothing at all, physical therapy, surgery, rest, or the use of various medications or drugs.

Even the best of veterinarians rarely has adequate time to go on at length in describing every diagnosis and its treatment. Good veterinarians are busy and generally the owner is provided enough knowledge to get the patient back to health, often without totally understanding the condition and why a particular medication is selected.

Treatments, especially medications (drugs), have evolved dramatically with the advancements of medicine. Some are more effective than others, while some are safer than others. The safest medication, however, is not always the best at curing the ailment.

The purpose of this book is to give dog owners a source of information about common veterinary drugs. In the past, few owners showed interest in the medications used to treat their pets. This is no longer true. Today's pet owners want to know more about their pet's ailments and treatments. At the Foster and Smith veterinary hospitals, we have always felt that the more educated the owner becomes, the quicker the pet will return to health. The reason is clear—the pet owner, not the veterinarian, provides most of the love and nurturing needed for recovery.

Medications, or drugs as they are commonly referred to, are usually prescribed to work one of two ways: they either alter the way the body functions or defend the patient from organisms that are attacking its body. Unfortunately, some medications also have unwanted actions, usually called adverse side effects. This book will take the reader through various body systems and describe the most common drugs used to keep the system functioning properly. When necessary, common side effects are also noted. There are medications not included in this text, but they are not commonly prescribed or are restricted to hospital usage.

Unfortunately, when one writes about medications, a certain level of technicality exists. To properly describe a medication, a book cannot necessarily be exciting to read. That's okay; this book is technical and is for the reader who desires more. By purchasing this book, you will have it in a time of need. Please let it serve as a reference, not to remove the need for a veterinarian, but as a source of knowledge. Together with your veterinarian, let this book help guide your pet to a healthy life as long as life is there.

PART I
An Overview of Medication Usage

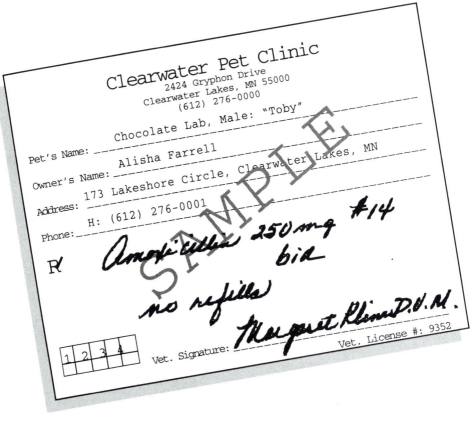

Figure 1-1: Prescription for 250mg Amoxicillin bid #14.

CHAPTER 1

The Selection of a Medication

After the owner has been questioned as to the animal's clinical signs or behavior, the patient examined, the blood tests and the X rays taken, and results received, hopefully the veterinarians will be able to make a diagnosis. In the initial stage, they may not be able to zero in on a single medical problem, but may have several different diagnoses in mind. If this is true, they may schedule additional tests or begin some sort of treatment aimed at the most likely problem. The animal's response to this therapy can further limit or define the exact cause of the illness.

Once the veterinarian has settled on some type of diagnosis, there is a wide range of potential treatments. Most treatments used in canine medicine are the same as those used for human patients. The surgical procedures are, with rare exceptions, identical. The same can be said for physical therapy, although that is used much more widely in human medicine. The majority of medications used in dogs are identical to those used in people. Sometimes they have the same brand names, while in other instances, even though their ingredients are identical, they go by completely different ones. And as would be expected, there are medications that are used only in either human or veterinary medicine. Additionally, within the field of veterinary medicine, some products are utilized in only one species while others are used in all. The veterinarian may therefore select the same or totally different medications than a human physician would for a similar condition. Almost all medications that are used both in human and veterinary medicine do, however, have totally different dosages in the two fields. As might be expected, the dosages for identical products often vary greatly when used for different species of animals.

Other differences in therapy between the veterinarian and the physician are brought on by the clinicians' respective abilities to communicate with their patients. In the case of a sprain or pulled muscle, the veterinarian will probably choose to do nothing more than rest the animal, restricting activity for a specific period of time. Treatment for the same condition in humans is different because the physician can communicate directly with the patient, explaining the injury and telling the patient to stay off the ankle. The hope is that the injured party complies. Because of this, the physician may also dispense or recommend a painkiller to bring additional comfort.

Since veterinarians cannot communicate in a straightforward fashion with dogs, the veterinarian may prefer that the patient feel some discomfort or pain, and may actually use it as a part of the treatment! This is because if the pain is completely eliminated with medication, the dog that sprained an ankle or pulled a muscle will probably return to normal activity levels, using the injured leg as before. Running after the paper boy with a sprained ankle could easily lead to a more serious injury. Painkillers and anti-inflammatories are very popular in veterinary medicine but, like many medications, they have their time and place.

Medical therapy may only be a part of the cure in some cases while in others it may constitute the entire treatment. In many situations, surgery, restricted activity, corrective diets, or physical therapy may be combined with the use of medications. The use of these other therapies may sometimes alter which or at what level medications are used. If a dog has an infection that developed into an abscess, it will usually be surgically opened and drained, and the animal put on antibiotics to wipe out any remaining bacterial organisms. If the infection has not yet localized or formed into an abscess, or if its location or the patient's medical condition or age prevent it from being surgically treated, a higher dose of the same antibiotics or additional medications may be used to correct the problem.

Regardless of circumstances, once the veterinarian decides on a medical therapy for an individual case, there are still many decisions to make: what should the drug accomplish, in what time frame, how it will be given, by whom, and what if any side effects will be allowed.

CLASSIFICATION OF MEDICATIONS BY ACTIVITY

When medications are administered to humans or animals, they have one of two major effects. One group of medications affects or modifies the patient and its systems' activities. In most cases these medications improve the abilities, or return to normal the functioning, of one or more of the body's organs or systems. These medicines are referred to as **pharmacotherapeutic agents;** they are the "body modifiers." Medications of a second group function to protect the patient by directing their therapeutic activity at another organism or abnormal cell type that has or may in the future take up residence on or in the patient's body. These are referred to as **chemotherapeutic agents,** the "body protectors." In the treatment of a single medical condition, the veterinarian may use different products from one or both categories simultaneously.

The body modifiers (pharmacotherapeutic agents) work on the patient directly. There are thousands of different medications in this category. They all alter the way the patient's body and its systems function. Usually this is done to correct something that is operating out of the normal range. There are many examples of these. If the heart has become weak and is failing, a pharmacotherapeutic agent such as **digitalis** would be used to strengthen it. If diarrhea has developed because the small intestine is irritated, thereby causing undigested food to move through the organ too rapidly, a pharmacotherapeutic agent such as **methscopolamine** may be used to slow down this section of the gastrointestinal tract. If a patient has developed epilepsy, a pharmacotherapeutic agent such as **phenobarbital** could be used to stabilize the neural system to prevent or decrease the severity or frequency of seizures. If a dog's thyroid gland is producing an inadequate amount of the thyroid hormone T4, resulting in a poor quality hair coat, breeding problems, obesity, and lethargy, then a pharmacotherapeutic agent such as the synthetic hormone **levothyroxine** will be given for the life of the animal to compensate for these deficiencies.

These are only a very few of the well known and commonly used pharmacotherapeutic agents. All the medications in this category are directed at the patient. They may be used for a very brief period, even a single dose, or they may be utilized throughout the life of the animal. They offer the patient no direct protection from potentially invasive foreign organisms such as fleas, worms, bacteria, etc. That is not their purpose. They are just as important as the chemotherapeutic medications, however, as they in some way affect the patient's physiology to return it to or maintain it within normal levels. Many animals would simply die or suffer severely without their use.

The second type of medications, the body protectors (chemotherapeutic agents), have their activity directed at unwanted organisms or cells that have made their way onto or within the patient's body. In canine medicine, we are constantly using these to eliminate such organisms as heartworms, roundworms, hookworms, fleas, ticks, mites, bacteria, viruses, fungi, etc. The list goes on and on. Chemotherapeutic medications may also be preventative, as they are used to protect the animal against future invasions of these same disease-causing organisms. And finally, the chemotherapeutic products are used to attack cells that have become foreign or harmful to a normally functioning body, as in the case of cancer.

As with the pharmacotherapeutic medications, the chemotherapeutic ones can be used for a very brief period of time, even a single dose, or they can be utilized for the life of the animal. Antibiotics, flea sprays and dips, worm tablets, topical antifungal creams, and some of the anticancer medications are just a few examples. In the life-and-death struggles of many dogs, they are no less important than the pharmacotherapeutic ones.

HOW PRODUCTS ARE LABELED AND SOLD

After the veterinarian has selected a medication and informed the client of the choice, the availability of the product to the pet owner may be restricted. That is to say, the product may be a prescription or *"legend"* product. These terms are synonymous and mean that the medication can only be purchased after the veterinarian has directed its usage. They carry on their label a statement or **"legend"** that in the case of a *veterinary product* reads *"Caution: Federal (USA) law restricts this drug to use by or on the order of a licensed veterinarian."* The labels of medications manufactured for the *human market* usually have the statement *"Caution: Federal law prohibits dispensing without prescription."* With some of these products, the veterinarian may dispense them directly to the pet owner without any mention of their restricted nature. In other instances, a prescription may be provided. This is a written form containing the pet's name, the owner's name, the medication, its quantity, the directions for use, and the signature of the veterinarian. This allows the pet owner to purchase the products wherever preferred. This can also be accomplished by the clinician phoning the prescription information directly to a particular pharmacy or other business with a pharmacy license. Figure 1-1 is a typical prescription written for fourteen 250mg amoxicillin capsules to be given twice daily.

The opposite of prescription or "legend" drugs are those sold **over-the-counter.** They're found on the shelves of every grocery, drug store, veterinary clinic, etc. The client simply walks into the store, makes a selection, buys it, and takes it home to use as desired. There will be directions on the bottle but no restriction as to its sale.

What determines whether a product is sold by a prescription or over-the-counter? When a new medication is first licensed and prepared for sale, how it will be marketed is determined by the actions of both the manufacturer and the federal government. Some companies may request that it be sold only by prescription to restrict their liability. If the government chooses to control the distribution or use of a potentially harmful product, it may require that the product be sold by prescription only. Later, after the medication has been used safely for several years, the legend may be removed, allowing it to be sold over-the-counter. A recent example would be cimetidine (Tagamet), the medication used to decrease acid production by the stomach in patients suffering from ulcers or similar disorders.

A sort of in-between ground occurs with certain veterinary products. They may be labeled "Sold only through licensed veterinarians," "Sales exclusively to graduate veterinarians," or in some similar manner. These statements usually signify a line of products where the manufacturer has decided to limit the channels of sale. In some cases, another line of products by the same manufacturer will have the same ingredients but be sold under a different name and found on the shelves of discount stores. Such marketing strategies are commonly used with flea and tick preparations.

Prescriptions also restrict the quantity the client can purchase at one time. A prescription is usually written with the intention that only one course of medicine will be used. They may, however, be labeled for a certain number of refills or noted with the letters "PRN." This means that the prescription can be refilled repeatedly at the client's request by the pharmacy without contacting the veterinarian. This is commonly done with medications that the animal will need over its entire life. Examples would be drugs to control seizures in the epileptic patient or hormonal supplementation in a dog suffering from hypothyroidism.

Regretfully, this process often restricts where the individual can purchase the medication and at what cost. Some prescription veterinary products are only sold by veterinarians. This obligates the client to purchase them through these channels. A veterinarian may prefer to sell human or veterinary products directly to the pet owner rather than write a prescription allowing the individual to buy the product at a pharmacy or other licensed business. Many veterinary clinics rely on the revenues earned from these products to contribute to their overall profit. Many pharmacies sell medications at very competitive prices that could potentially save the individual significant sums of money. If veterinarians refuse to provide a prescription and demand to sell the product themselves, the client may be spending much more money than is necessary. The owner of the dog being placed on a prescription product has the right to request a written prescription so that he or she may purchase the product wherever he or she may choose. Most veterinarians will happily do this. In some states, they are required by law to honor such a request.

By law, a prescription can only be given by the veterinarian who has examined or has personal knowledge of the patient and the case. A pet owner cannot call relatives or friends who happen to be veterinarians and expect them to legally supply a prescription. If they haven't seen or examined the animal, they cannot prescribe these restricted products.

Drugs, whether they are prescription or over-the-counter, are often available in two forms: **brand name** or **generic.** In the last few decades, generic substitutes for the often more expensive brand name products have been seen for everything from breakfast cereal to cancer drugs. Why do both forms exist in medicine? In some cases, a company that manufactures a certain drug may choose to sell the product both under its brand name and in a cheaper generic form to capture a wider market. The federal government strictly requires that both forms comply exactly with the label. In other instances, the less expensive generic form will be manufactured and sold by a totally different company. The makeup of the two products must still rigidly comply with the federal standards. In this second case, however, the original developer or manufacturer may have lost the patent rights. In medicine, the holder of the original patent is protected for a period of years, usually seventeen, from any other company manufacturing and selling the product without their written permission. The theory is that this enables pharmaceutical firms to spend large sums of money in research and development of new medications, since they are protected and can recoup these investments. However, after this period other firms are allowed to manufacture and sell the medication in an attempt to keep the cost of these products as low as possible for the consumer.

The obvious question for dog owners is whether they can or should request generic medications, be they prescription or over-the-counter. In most veterinary and human clinics today, a major portion of the medications lining the shelves are already generics. This is especially true of orally administered products. Examples would be antibiotics, anti-inflammatories, anticonvulsants, and hormone replacements. Still, there are many times when clients can make significant savings by requesting generic products, especially if they are taking a written prescription to a discount pharmacy. In the authors' experience, with the exception of some heart stimulants or hormonal products such as those used in hypothyroid patients, little difference has been found in the outcome of cases when generics were used in place of brand name products.

WHAT THE PRESCRIPTION MEANS TO THE DOG OWNER

Importantly, prescriptions define the quantity of medication to be dispensed and therefore to be used. With rare exceptions, when a prescription medication is dispensed, it is assumed that *all* will be used. If there are fourteen capsules in the bottle, it means that all fourteen should be used unless problems occur or other directions are given. Plan to use the entire quantity. However, if the animal fails to improve or abnormal signs are noted, it is the responsibility of the owner to contact the veterinarian and describe these developments.

The owner of the dog, the one actually paying the bills, has the right to request a prescription so that medication may be purchased in the most economical way. Additionally, they have the same right to request a generic substitute or at least ask if one exists for the product utilized.

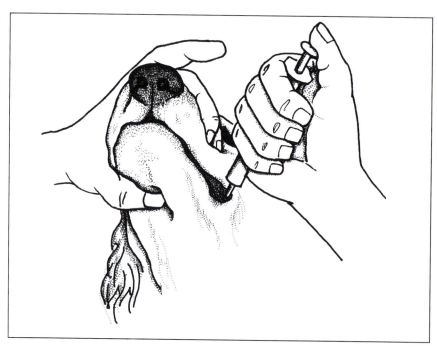

Figure 2-1: Liquid medication being administered in cheek pouch.

CHAPTER 2

Route of Administration

How a particular medication will be administered to the animal will sometimes be decided by the veterinarian, but in some cases the choice of product may dictate how it can be given. Medications can either be applied **topically** or given **systemically.**

Topically means that the product is applied to the outer or external surfaces of the body. This may be done to the surface of the skin, within the ear canal, on the surface of the eye, within one of the openings of the body, etc. Topical medications include such preparations as creams, lotions, liquid sprays and dips, powders, and liniments. They come packaged in tubes, bottles, canisters, and other types of applicators. Most dog owners have used them in the treatment of ear infections, skin abrasions, or flea and tick problems.

Topical medications may exert all of their therapeutic activity directly on the surface of the skin, or they may be formulated in such a way that their active ingredients are absorbed into the body. Most dog owners believe that topical preparations are safer because they do not get "inside of their pet's body." This is not true of most topical preparations, as they are absorbed through the skin and enter deeper structures. A portion of topical medications will usually enter the bloodstream and be carried throughout the animal's body. Examples of those that are applied on the body's surface but penetrate the skin and reach the deeper areas are most of the antibiotics and steroids found in ear, eye, and skin preparations used to control infections and inflammations. Almost all the active ingredients of the flea and tick medications, and to a lesser extent portions of the moisturizing and soothing skin preparations, are absorbed through the skin to some degree. There are also products known as liniments that are designed to carry other substances through the skin. These are typically applied over irritated joints or muscles.

Systemic administration of a medication means that the drug is given internally. This may be accomplished in several different ways. It can be taken **orally** or **parenterally**. **Parenteral** means it enters the body by a route other than through the intestinal tract. In the dog, these are given by injection or as an inhalant (as is the case with many anesthetic agents). Depending on how it is given and the properties of the medication, a drug may remain restricted to certain areas or spread throughout the body.

Oral administration is the preferred method when a dog must be treated at home. In most instances, it is easier for owners to give a product orally than it is to give an injection. Many times it can simply be mixed with food. Most oral medications pass through the stomach into the small intestine, where they are absorbed by the blood vessels lining that organ. From this point, the product is transported into the larger blood vessels and then distributed throughout the body.

Oral products have other important advantages, the first of which is cost. A single dose of most medications, be it a chemotherapeutic one such as an antibiotic or a pharmacotherapeutic product like a heart drug, is much cheaper in the oral form rather than as an injection. Tablets, capsules, and oral liquids are much less expensive and easier to manufacture and package than when produced in an injectable form. They do not have to be sterile, rarely require refrigeration, and usually last much longer in storage.

Oral products have additional advantages for the patient. Undesirable reactions can occur with any medication but are much less common when the product is given orally versus given as an injection. Additionally, after a single administration, medications given orally generally have a longer effective time period in the body than injections. Injections tend to enter the blood system quickly and are therefore excreted from the body in a shorter time. Also, if the veterinarian wants the medication to function within the gastrointestinal tract, oral administration is usually preferred. There are numerous useful and very safe products that are never absorbed into the body after oral administration; these remain in the gastrointestinal tract where they carry out their function. Examples of these would be many of the wormers or certain antibiotics. If given by injection, they would not be able to reach the area where their activity was required and in many instances could cause toxic side effects.

There are some disadvantages to the oral route for systemic administration. Some have to do with the product and others with the health of the animal. As stated, certain medications cannot be absorbed by the animal's gastrointestinal tract. While at times this can be used to the advantage of the clinician, in other cases it is a problem. Many antibiotics never reach the bloodstream if given orally, but rather pass out in the stool. An example would be the antibiotic gentamicin. Also, the time it takes for a medication to start working after oral administration is always longer than when given as an injection.

Stressed or unhealthy animals are rarely good candidates for oral medication. Sometimes they have difficulty absorbing these medications. In some severely debilitated animals, the GI tract of the patients may "shut down" and not function at all. In these cases, little or no absorption of the intestinal contents can occur. Additionally, if a patient is suffering from a gastrointestinal upset such as vomiting or diarrhea, the medication may not be in these areas of the body long enough for absorption to occur.

GIVING ORAL MEDICATIONS

As stated, oral medications come in liquid, capsule, or tablet form and each can be given in different ways. There may be restrictions with any form. Some can be given with food and some cannot. Some can be given on a full stomach and some cannot. Some cannot be given with certain kinds of food such as dairy products; with other medications, it may be better to give them with dairy products. With some there may be a period of fasting required before or after administration, but with most this is not important. Some tablets or capsules should not be broken, as they are coated to decrease irritation to the mouth or stomach or to hide a bad taste. All these restrictions are to ensure that the medication is tolerated by the patient and absorbed correctly.

Liquids are probably the easiest to administer. They are usually flavored so that the dog at least will not dislike the taste. They can often be mixed with food. Small quantities can be dropped or squirted into the mouth over the tongue with some success.

However, it's usually better, especially with large quantities, to tilt the dog's head back, hold its mouth shut, and squirt or pour the solution into the pouch between its teeth and cheek. (See Figure 2-1.) With the pet's mouth held shut, the tongue will not be able to flip back and forth, spraying medicine over the owner and area. It's also best to do this on the left side of the dog's mouth as this facilitates passage into the esophagus.

Capsules or tablets can often be mixed with food. Tablets can be crushed or capsules opened and the powder mixed with the food to better facilitate hiding the medication. To administer pills or capsules to the dog without crushing or opening them, it will help to put a small quantity of butter, margarine, or oil on them so they slide down the throat easier without sticking to the inner surface of the dog's mouth.

The administration of tablets or capsules to a dog can be very easy or, with less compliant dogs, a test of will and courage. Some dogs take them as if they were a treat, while others must be tempted. When giving tablets or capsules directly, first open the dog's mouth wide. This is easiest if the thumb gently presses the upper lip against the upper teeth and roof of the dog's mouth. This decreases the chance of being bitten. (See Figure 2-2.) Then the lubricated pill or capsule is pushed over the back of the dog's tongue. Quickly close the mouth, hold it shut, and encourage the pet to swallow. This can be done by either rubbing its throat or blowing in its nose. Watch closely to ensure that the animal swallows. It is a good idea to reopen the mouth to make sure the medication isn't visible.

The injectable administration of a medication is typically restricted to use within a clinic environment. However, many owners do administer injections. This may be for medical treatments, routine vaccinations, or daily therapy (as is the case for a diabetic receiving insulin). Injections permit the most rapid onset of action of the medication. However, exactly how the injection is given has a great effect on just how fast the drug starts to function. Injections can be given through three different routes or sites: intravenously (**IV**), intramuscularly (**IM**) or subcutaneously (**SQ**).

Medications given through the IV method work the fastest because they are deposited directly into the bloodstream and quickly transported throughout the body to the intended site of their activity. Injections given IM are fairly rapid in their onset of action.

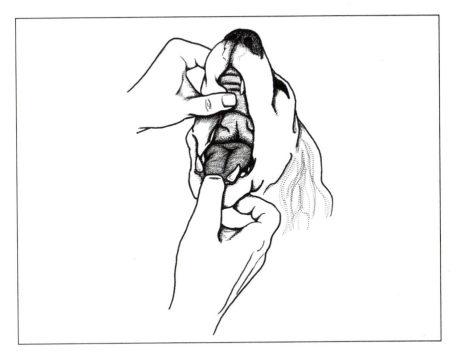

Figure 2-2: Holding mouth open.

This is because muscles have numerous blood vessels coursing through their mass, supplying these active tissues with oxygen and nutrients. The drug is rapidly picked up by these blood vessels following an IM injection. The injections taking the longest to become effective are SQ. The subcutaneous tissue does not have a rich blood supply and it therefore takes longer for the medication to make its way into a blood vessel. This slower absorption in IM or SQ sites is sometimes potentiated further with some products that use a "slow release" carrier for the actual medication. The release of the product can then be extended over weeks or months.

In which injection site a product is given and how fast it works is also affected by how it is formulated. Injectable products are usually water or oil based. Oil-based ones cannot be given directly into a blood vessel by the IV route because the oil would not dissolve and could clog blood vessels throughout the body. This could easily kill the patient if the affected vessels were in the brain, heart, lungs, or other critical tissues. When oil-based products are given through the IM or SQ routes, the medication is absorbed slowly. Most

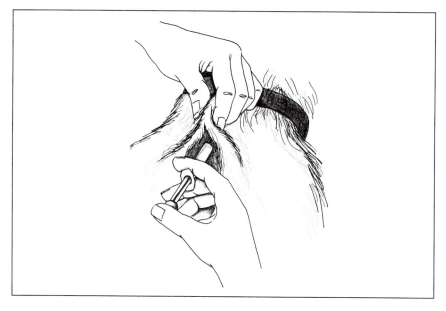

Figure 2-3: Subcutaneous injection.

water-based products can be injected at any site and work faster than the oil-based ones, as it is easier for them to dissolve and make their way into the blood vessels.

Whether an injection is given IV, IM, or SQ also depends on properties of the medication. Some are very irritating to the body's tissues. This may be because of their pH (i.e., they may be strong acids or bases) or some other caustic property. Those that are severely irritating must usually be given IV, slowly. This allows them to be diluted by the blood. In the muscle or subcutaneous areas, these medications might result in abscesses or chemical burning.

Dog owners, to their surprise, rarely have a problem giving injections. In our experience, many clients have done this for daily administration of insulin to a diabetic pet, routine vaccinations, or even occasional medical treatments such as antibiotics.

Subcutaneous injections are the easiest to administer. They are the easiest on the pet also, as they are usually painless. Probably the best site for SQ injections is in the loose skin over the neck and shoulders. The skin and hair can be disinfected with alcohol or another disinfectant. Remember, however, it takes alcohol and disinfectants a few minutes to kill or inactivate bacteria and other organisms. The wiping of the skin and hair coat is probably done more for appearance than actual benefit. The skin is then picked

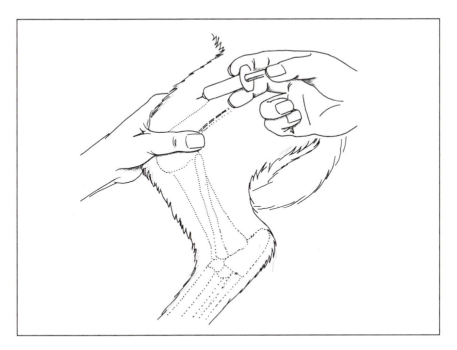

Figure 2-4: Hind leg injection site.

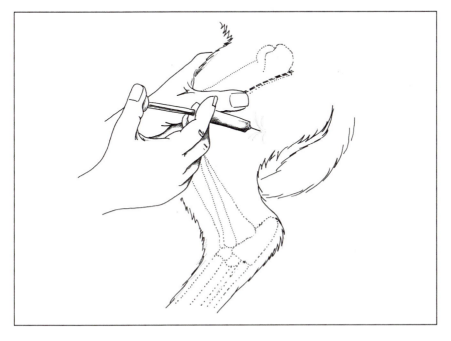

Figure 2-5: Directing needle caudally.

up between the thumb and forefinger like a tent. As it is lifted, a small dimple forms below the thumb and finger. The needle is quickly placed in this area (Figure 2-3). The plunger is then pulled back to ensure that the end of the needle is not in a blood vessel. This is called **aspiration.** If blood appears in the syringe, the needle is withdrawn from the animal and a second location is tried. If no blood appears, the plunger is pushed into the syringe and the medication is administered. The needle and syringe are then withdrawn from the skin.

Intramuscular injections are usually given in the muscle of the hind leg. This can be done in front of or behind the large bone in the upper portion of the leg (Figure 2-4). The front portion is the safest, as damage to a nerve cannot be caused at this site. If one chooses to give the injection in the back portion of the leg, then the thumb should be placed behind the bone and the needle directed backwards from there (Figure 2-5). Regardless of the site, after the skin and hair are disinfected, the needle is passed through the skin into the muscle. Aspiration is done as with the SQ injection. If blood enters the syringe, then the needle is withdrawn and another site used. When no blood appears, the plunger is pushed into the syringe, administering the medication. The needle and syringe are then withdrawn.

Intravenous injections are usually only done by trained personnel. These injections are typically given in the large blood vessels of the front leg or neck. The vessel is held off with a tourniquet or thumb. The hair and skin are disinfected and the needle placed into the vein. Aspiration is done, but this time blood *should* come back into the syringe. If it does not, then the needle is redirected into the vein. The plunger is pushed into the body of the syringe, dispensing the medication. The needle and syringe are then withdrawn. Sometimes intravenous injections are administered through an IV fluid line.

How a medication is formulated, how it is administered, and how it will affect the patient are all related. The owner of a dog may not choose which particular medication is used or how it is administered, but should know that there are differences which affect whether the pet can be medicated at home or will have to remain in a hospital. One should also be able to consistently administer the medication when the dog is in one's care.

CHAPTER 3

Distribution of Medications Once They Are Within the Body

Once within the body, drugs are predominantly transported to various areas by the bloodstream. This usually allows the medication to get to the specific area where treatment is needed. With most drugs, however, it should be understood that the medication will be found in almost every area of the body whether the preparation is needed there or not. Because of this, the quantity of a drug given is higher than that actually directed for use within a specific tissue. For example, if an antibiotic such as amoxicillin is being used to treat pneumonia, there is a specified dosage that will be used. It should be remembered, however, that probably only about 20 percent of this actual quantity will go into the lungs; the majority will be distributed within the other tissues of the body. Therefore, *when we treat one area, we usually treat the entire body.*

There are exceptions to this, as certain areas require medications to have special properties to reach them. An example would be the central nervous system, i.e., the brain and spinal cord. There exists a "blood-brain barrier" that prevents many medications from entering these areas. The blood vessels and membranes of the central nervous system are different from those found elsewhere in the body and passage through their walls is more limited. The size and various chemical properties of the actual molecules of the medication determine whether or not passage can occur. Of course, smaller molecules pass more easily. Also, fat soluble products gain access more readily to the central nervous system than water soluble ones.

ALTERATIONS OF SOME MEDICATIONS
WITHIN THE BODY

Topical preparations are formulated to function immediately after application without the body altering them in any way. Most medications are already in the correct form to be effective whether they make their way into the body by absorption through the skin or via the oral or injectable routes. Others must be altered, usually through chemical reactions, before they can function as intended. In some cases they must be changed so that they can enter the area where they are targeted to act. Others are simply changed by the patient's body into a more chemically or biologically active form. The majority of these reactions that transform medications into effective therapeutic forms occur in the liver. There can be found a wide range of enzymes to expedite these conversions within the cells. To be effective, these medications therefore require that the patient have a normal, healthy, functioning liver. Additionally, some medications may increase or decrease the rate at which these reactions within the liver take place. By doing this, these medications sometimes alter the dosages of other drugs.

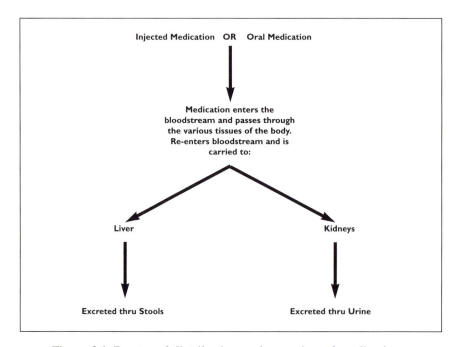

Figure 3-1: Routes of distribution and excretion of medications.

EXCRETION FROM THE BODY

The portion of a topical medication that is not absorbed and remains on the surface of the body simply wears off over a period of time. Some medications may evaporate (as do some flea and tick preparations), but most come off due to normal abrasion. Drugs that have entered the body are eliminated by a process of one or more steps. Some pass through and exit unchanged, leaving the body in the exact same chemical form as when they entered it. This could occur via the urine or stool. Others must first be metabolized, changed, or broken down before they can be excreted. In most cases, but not all, this breakdown occurs through chemical processes inside the various cells of the body. The most common site for this is within the liver.

As stated, medications are usually eliminated from the body through either the urine or the stool. Medications or their metabolized portions are carried to the kidneys via the bloodstream, passing through various microscopic structures, and are expelled via the urine. Others will pass through the liver, be excreted into the bile, pass through the bile duct into the intestines, and be eliminated with the stool. Some medications can alter the rate at which excretion from the liver or kidneys takes place. For example, a diuretic that increases urine production can speed up the excretion of a medication by the kidney and therefore alter its dosage or frequency of administration. The same is true of other medications that speed up or slow down liver metabolism. They alter the dosage rates of products that are normally eliminated by the liver.

The method of excretion can be utilized therapeutically. If a bacterial infection is present in the bladder—i.e., a **cystitis**—then an antibiotic that passes out through the urine unchanged can be chosen. High concentrations of the product will be deposited with the urine directly into the bladder where the disease-causing organisms reside. Medications that are taken orally but are not absorbed through the intestinal wall will remain in the gastrointestinal tract and pass out in the stool. They can be used to treat bacterial or parasitic infections of the intestinal tract.

It must be remembered that the speed with which a product is metabolized or expelled from the body affects how long the medication is at effective levels and how frequently it must be given. These factors are always taken into consideration when dosages are determined or altered.

SUMMARY

As you will see as we make our way through this book, the veterinarian has a wide range of potential medications to choose from when treating an individual dog. Our goal will be to help you understand the medication, why the selection was made, how it can be given, its effects on the dog or the microorganism against which its activity may be directed, and how it is metabolized and eliminated. As an owner you may or may not help in the initial selection of a particular medication, but you should understand its role and any potential side effects.

P A R T   I I

The Chemotherapeutic Medications

THE BODY PROTECTORS

When most owners hear the term **chemotherapeutic** or **chemotherapy,** they usually think only of the treatment of cancer. While this is not necessarily incorrect, the phrase **chemotherapeutic agents** includes all medications whose activity is directed against unwanted cells or organisms that are found on or within the patient's body. These could range from fleas to bacteria to cancer cells and everything in between. Chemotherapeutic medications, although they may and often do cause unwanted side effects, are not intended to affect or alter the activity of the patient's body but rather to protect it from other potentially harmful organisms or cells. They are called the "body protectors." Pharmacotherapeutic drugs, the other major classification of medications, have their activity directed at the patient and alter the way the body functions. They are the "body modifiers."

Chemotherapeutic medications are routinely used in canine medicine. It is this group of drugs that is most commonly administered to the animal by the owner. They can be divided into the following groups: antimicrobials (which include antibiotics and other antibacterial drugs, antifungals and antivirals), antiparasitics, and anticancer medications. These may be taken orally, given by injection, or applied topically. They may be used for a brief period of time or for the life of the dog. Additionally, they may be used as preventatives, hopefully eliminating some future problem, or as a treatment for a current one.

Antimicrobials are often characterized by their action. Sometimes a suffix is added to the word to better define this action. For example, a drug may be said to be **bacteriostatic,** i.e., one that slows down or inhibits the growth of a bacteria; or **bactericidal,** i.e., one that kills bacteria. Some are described as **broad spectrum,** i.e., those that affect a wide range of microorganisms with different characteristics; or **narrow spectrum,** i.e., those that affect only a few different microorganisms, all with very similar properties.

Although only one chemotherapeutic agent is usually used at any one time, there are terms used to describe their effect on each other's action if two or more of these medications are used simultaneously. If a medication is referred to as being **synergistic** with another, this means that its activity is helpful or additive in nature when the two are used together. It is said that medications are **antagonistic** to each other if their mechanisms of action retard or inhibit each other's ability to function as intended. If two or more drugs are used at the same time but they in no way affect each other's functions, it is said they are **indifferent** to each other.

It must not be forgotten that whether a medication such as an antibiotic is classified as bacteriostatic or bactericidal, narrow or broad spectrum, synergistic or antagonistic, in most instances the success of these medications requires some participation of the patient's own immune system. They may only reduce the microorganism's development, growth, or total numbers enough so that the patient's own defenses can eliminate the infectious organism. This is especially true with medications carrying the "-static" ending.

One last factor must be understood when considering the use of antimicrobials, and that is the combination of **resistance** and **sensitivity. Resistance** can best be described as the ability or property of a microorganism that allows it to be basically unaffected by a chemotherapeutic medication. The drug is then ineffective against that potentially harmful microbe. There can be different levels of resistance; it is not always an all-or-nothing situation. In some instances, a medication may not be as effective as is normally expected but still may have some effect on the microbe. Conversely, a microorganism is said to be **sensitive** to a particular medication if the drug either inhibits its growth and action or kills it.

Additionally, resistance can be **natural** or **acquired. Natural resistance** is when certain properties or lack of certain properties of a particular microbial organism or cell prevent specific medications from affecting that organism or cell's life or activity. For example, let's say that a new antibiotic was developed that killed all bacteria with an XYZ molecule in the cell wall. For the sake of discussion, the antibiotic attached to and dissolved the XYZ molecule, thereby rupturing the cell wall and killing the bacteria. Therefore, other bacterial species that did not have the XYZ molecule in their cell walls would have a natural resistance to the new drug. The new medication would be totally ineffective against these bacteria.

Acquired resistance describes a situation when a microorganism that has been sensitive to a particular medication somehow alters its properties or structure such that the drug affects it no longer, or to a lesser degree. This generally occurs over time, especially when the microbial species is in prolonged contact with the medication. Most microorganisms reproduce rapidly with very short periods between generations. Additionally, when an infection does occur within a patient's body, there are usually millions and millions of organisms present. Such huge populations have a wide range of characteristics. Resistance can occur if a mutation occurs that now protects the microbe from the drug or if a very small percentage of the population has a characteristic that is protective in nature. Those that are spared the activity of the drug rapidly increase in numbers, replacing those that were affected by its mechanism of action. In the above example, if a mutation occurs such that the bacterial species no longer has the XYZ molecule in its cell wall or in some way hides it from the drug, it has developed resistance to the new antibiotic. Another common cause of acquired resistance occurs when bacteria basically take the offensive against the antibacterial medication and produce their own enzymes that break down or inactivate the drug. These and other methods of acquired resistance often do not take a long time to develop. They can take place over a period of only a few days.

A common scenario would be when a veterinarian prescribes a two-week course of an antibiotic in an attempt to eliminate an infection. During the first few days of treatment all seems to be going well, with the patient improving. However, after four or five days the bacteria develop a resistance to the medication and the infection returns to its previous level. In other cases, the bacteria may already have a natural or acquired resistance before the medication is started, and what was assumed to be appropriate therapy has no effect at all.

Microorganismal resistance to medications occurs all the time. Today, many veterinarians and other members of the health community are concerned about this phenomenon. Older antibiotics have lost much of their effectiveness because many bacterial species have been exposed to these medications for such a long period of time that many are developing resistance to them. This is why many health professionals want to see the use of antimicrobial medications restricted and used only when absolutely necessary.

SUMMARY

These terms and principles apply to all the chemotherapeutic medications. Whether we are discussing antibiotics, flea sprays, or cancer therapy, the same ideas and principles must be taken into consideration.

CHAPTER 4

The Fight Against Bacteria and Related Organisms— Antimicrobials

There are several different kinds of disease-causing microorganisms that affect the dog. Among those within this category and covered in this chapter are **bacteria, mycoplasma, chlamydia,** and **rickettsia.** Some microbiologists consider them all bacteria but most separate them because of their differences in morphology, activity, and susceptibility to medications.

Bacteria are common, tiny, microscopic organisms, many of which cause serious diseases in dogs. They can best be described as one-celled, but containing genetic material that allows their reproduction through simple binary fission. They may live free within the environment or within another organism. While in another animal or plant, they may live within their host's cells or float freely within the fluid between cells or in compartments such as the bladder or stomach.

They can be anywhere within an animal. While it is true that probably only a small percentage of the total number of bacterial species actually cause any form of medical disorder, their names and the diseases they are responsible for are heard every day. **Strep throat, tetanus, leptospirosis,** and **"staph"** are a just a few examples. Additionally, many medical conditions in dogs that can be caused by many different kinds of organisms are most typically brought on by bacterial species. Common examples would be pneumonia, bladder infections, diarrhea, skin infections, etc. Another condition that commonly requires treatment of a bacterial problem is when an infection is actually secondary to that of another kind of microorganism. For example, in the dog, viral pneumonia commonly occurs with or is followed by a secondary bacterial infection of the lungs.

Bacteria can be treated with any of the antibiotics or antibacterials discussed in this chapter. Among the most commonly used in canine medicine today are amoxicillin (one of the penicillins), Baytril (one of the quinolones), Tribrissen or Primor (members of the sulfonamide group), and tetracycline. While there may be hundreds of antibiotics available today, most veterinarians use only a few.

Rickettsia and **chlamydia** are smaller than bacteria and are unique in that they must live within the cells of other organisms. That is, they are not free-living within the environment. They have cell walls and divide or multiply by simple binary fission. They commonly cause infections associated with blood cells or the respiratory and ocular systems. They are treated with some of the same medications used to treat bacteria. Products that can be used against either rickettsial or chlamydial organisms would be some of the tetracyclines, macrolides, sulfonamides, quinolones, or chloramphenicol. Of these, members of the tetracycline family are most commonly used.

Mycoplasma are even smaller than the rickettsial or chlamydial organisms. They have no cell walls and may be free-living. Mycoplasmal organisms often cause respiratory, genitourinary, and ocular infections. These infections can be treated with some of the macrolides, aminoglycosides, lincosamides, tetracyclines, quinolones, and chloramphenicol.

To treat bacteria, mycoplasma, chlamydia, or rickettsia, an antibiotic, antimicrobial, or antibacterial can be used. The terms for these medications are often used interchangeably but some differences do exist. Remember that an antibiotic is a substance produced by one microorganism that inhibits the growth of or kills another. An antibacterial is a substance that inhibits or kills bacteria. It may or may not be an antibiotic. Some antibacterials such as the sulfas are not antibiotics but are produced by manufacturing processes. Antimicrobials are substances used against any microbial organism such as bacteria, yeasts, parasites, etc. They could be antibiotics, other antibacterials, antiviral drugs, etc.

There are basically *four* different types of **antibacterial medications** that can be used in veterinary medicine today: **antibiotics,**

sulfonamides, nitrofurans, and **quinolones.** Of these, the sulfon-amides and antibiotics account for over 95 percent of all antibacter-ial therapy in canine medicine. The use of the quinolones has increased dramatically in the past few years. Most of the nitrofurans have been removed from the market in the last few years and there-fore will not be covered.

ANTIBIOTICS

Antibiotic therapy really started with the discovery of **penicillin.** It was not originally manufactured or perfected with the intention of treating bacterial diseases. Rather, it was observed that a certain fungus had the ability to prevent bacterial growth in its vicinity. Through research, it was found that a particular chemical substance produced by the fungus was responsible for this inhibition of the bacteria. This was penicillin.

Antibiotics are, by definition, a substance produced by one microorganism that retards or kills another microorganism. Today's pharmaceutical firms are still discovering new antibiotics by testing soil, compost heaps, and any other environment that contains naturally occurring microorganismal species. Originally, once an antibiotic had been isolated, these firms had to grow cultures of the microorganism responsible for producing more of the substance. While this is still done today, once found in nature many antibiotics are produced artificially in the laboratory. Sometimes their natu-rally occurring structure is altered to increase strength or decrease toxic side effects.

There are *several different groups of antibiotics* used in canine medi-cine. They have different mechanisms of action, are effective against different kinds of bacteria, may be distributed in the body differently, may cause unwanted side effects, and can be eliminated from the body in a variety of ways. The selection of an antibiotic depends on *all* of these factors.

Since the selection of an antibiotic is usually done when an infec-tion is present, probably the most important criterion is that the medication be effective against that particular microorganism. To do this, the veterinarian will do laboratory tests to determine the type of bacterial organism that is present. These tests can be very complex, identifying the exact species of bacteria present, but this degree of accuracy usually requires several days. More commonly

only a simple Gram stain is done on the bacteria. This is done by first isolating the bacteria from the infection. This might be from urine in the case of a bladder infection, sputum that is brought up with coughing in pneumonia, a pimple-like structure filled with pus in a skin infection, etc. The organisms are mixed with a stain, specifically a Gram stain, and then examined under a microscope. The sample's appearance will tell the veterinarian the shape of the bacteria and whether or not the Gram stain attaches to the bacterial organism. The shape will be defined in terms such as "rod" or "spherical," and as to the stain, they will be either Gram-positive (those to which the stain attached) or Gram-negative (those where the stain did not attach). The shape and staining characteristics often tell the veterinarian what type of bacterial species is present and give some indication of which antibacterial should be used.

To better help a veterinarian decide exactly which antibacterial should be used, a "culture and sensitivity" may also be performed. This is done by taking the previously isolated bacteria and growing it on a culture medium within a petri dish. On the same surface of this medium are placed small circular pieces of paper, each containing minute concentrations of different antibiotics. The culture plate is examined approximately twenty-four hours later. Antibiotics that are effective against the organism in question will prevent bacterial growth around the paper. (See Figure 4-1.) Although simplified here, this process allows the veterinarian to select an antibacterial medication to which the bacteria is sensitive.

Veterinarians sometimes choose to combine two or more antibacterials simultaneously on the same patient. Combination therapy is done when the activities or mechanisms of action of the two medications allow them to work synergistically. This means that their individual abilities to eliminate or control the infection are enhanced when they work together. Which medications can be effectively used together is not found from the culture and sensitivity results but rather from an understanding of the properties of the different antibacterials.

THE PENICILLIN ANTIBIOTICS

This chapter started with discussion of the penicillins, not because they were the first discovered but because they are probably the most commonly used in canine medicine today. They are a very safe and effective group. Included in this group are familiar names such

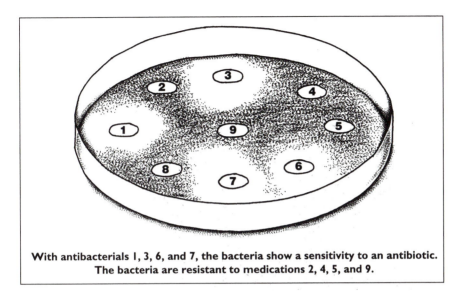

With antibacterials 1, 3, 6, and 7, the bacteria show a sensitivity to an antibiotic. The bacteria are resistant to medications 2, 4, 5, and 9.

Figure 4-1.

as **penicillin, penicillin G, ampicillin, amoxicillin, hetacillin, car-benicillin, cloxacillin,** etc. They come in oral and injectable forms and are sold under a wide range of trade names and in many generic formulations. Some are isolated from natural cultures while others are synthesized in the laboratory.

The action of the penicillin group when used at recommended dosage levels is bactericidal, i.e., these antibiotics actually kill bacterial organisms. As the population of bacteria multiplies, these medications function by preventing them from forming cell walls around their internal structures. Without a complete and functional cell wall, these bacteria die. While the original penicillin was effective only against the Gram-positive organisms, the newer ones such as ampicillin, amoxicillin, cloxacillin, etc., are much more broad spectrum, affecting Gram-positive and Gram-negative forms. Bacteria commonly have or develop resistance against the penicillins. Although this can occur through several different mechanisms, most commonly the bacteria produce an enzyme called B-lactamase that breaks down the antibiotic molecule.

Once inside the body, whether taken orally or by injection, penicillins are picked up by the bloodstream and carried through most areas of the body. Under normal situations they do not pass through the blood-brain barrier into the central nervous system, but if this structure is inflamed or diseased, they do pass into these areas. After circulating through the body and reaching therapeutic levels in most areas, the various antibiotics within the penicillin group are excreted by the kidneys through the urine. The medications are not altered or metabolized by the body in any way. They leave the body with the same molecular structure with which they entered.

The penicillins and the various synthetics in this group are widely used in veterinary medicine for many reasons. They are safe and effective against many different bacterial species, but additionally, they require no metabolism to a more active form as is common with some antibacterials. This means that sick or debilitated animals or those with poor liver function (the site of most such metabolism) tolerate the medications very well. They can be used on anything from newborn puppies to very old dogs. They are used to treat infections throughout the body. This includes all soft tissue areas including the central nervous system. They are preferred for urinary tract infections, where the organisms present are sensitive to the antibiotic excreted unchanged *into* these areas. They are popular in mastitis cases in lactating females. Most of the penicillins will pass into the milk in these cases; many veterinarians welcome this, as the antibiotic can be carried into the puppies that may have consumed the same bacteria. The penicillins are sometimes used in combination with other antibacterials belonging to the aminoglycoside group, such as gentamicin or streptomycin. Certain members of these groups work synergistically, greatly increasing their collective effect on the bacteria.

Serious side effects are very, very rare with members of the penicillin group. Penicillin allergies or reactions are common in humans but very rare in the dog. When they do occur, usually only a mild rash or fever is noted. Occasionally, long term oral use of such members of this group as ampicillin or amoxicillin may alter the normal bacterial flora of the gastrointestinal tract, leading to diarrhea. This is uncommon and the animal usually returns to normal when the medication is withdrawn from use.

THE CEPHALOSPORIN ANTIBIOTICS

The **cephalosporins** have many similarities with the penicillins. They are also bactericidal, exerting their action against the production of the cell wall by the bacteria. Commonly used members of this group include **cephalexin** (Keflex), **cefadroxil** (Cefa-Tabs), **cefaclor**

(Ceclor), and **cefixime** (Cefixime). These medications are available in several oral and injectable forms. As with the penicillins, the cephalosporins have undergone continual improvement since their initial discovery in the mid-1960s. They have always been considered broad spectrum antibiotics, but the range of effectiveness continues to expand. The first ones were predominately effective against Gram-positive organisms with only marginal activity against the Gram-negative ones. Those developed in the last few years are exceptionally effective against both types of bacteria. Bacterial resistance to the cephalosporins does occur but much less frequently than is seen with the penicillins.

Once administered orally or by injection, the cephalosporins are spread throughout most areas of the patient's body through the bloodstream. Effective concentrations are found in all tissues except those protected by the blood-brain barrier. Unlike the penicillins, they are prevented from entering the central nervous system even when these areas are inflamed. There are few food types that affect the absorption of these medications when they are given orally.

Most of the antibiotics in this group do not need to be metabolized or changed to a more active form. They are administered in the basic form, which is also the active antibacterial structure. A few do require some modification by the liver to become more effective. As with the penicillins, most cephalosporins are excreted unchanged through the kidneys and into the urine.

The cephalosporins are used to treat a wide range of bacterial infections. One factor that often limits their use is their expense. It is usually three to four times more expensive to treat an animal with this group of antibiotics as it is to use one of the newer broad spectrum penicillins. Still, they are very safe and effective, especially against some of the more difficult-to-treat bacterial species such as *Pseudomonas*. Almost all soft and bony tissues can be treated by these antibiotics, and since they are excreted into the urine unaltered, they are often used to treat bladder infections. Their antibacterial activity works synergistically when used in combination with the aminoglycosides.

While the cephalosporins would be considered very safe in the dog, some reactions have been reported. A few animals have displayed hypersensitivity (allergic) reactions such as skin rashes and mild fevers. It is interesting to note that animals that react this way often have a similar response to the penicillins and vice versa.

A very few patients treated with the cephalosporins have been reported to experience toxic side effects associated with kidney function. Because of this, cephalosporins are usually not used in animals with kidney failure or impaired kidney function.

THE AMINOGLYCOSIDES

This group of medications can be used in simultaneously with the penicillins and cephalosporins, but the **aminoglycosides** are very different from these previously discussed antibiotics. Some examples of antibiotics in this group are **gentamicin, kanamycin, neomycin, amikacin, tobramycin, streptomycin,** and **dihydrostreptomycin.** They can be found in topical, oral, and injectable forms. Most topical and oral forms are usually combination products containing one or more additional medications.

The aminoglycosides are bactericidal. They enter the bacterial cell and prevent it from multiplying or surviving by inhibiting protein synthesis. Although there is some variation in the group, they are generally considered broad spectrum antibiotics, effective against some Gram-positive and most Gram-negative organisms. They also can be used to treat infections caused by mycoplasmal organisms. Even though these are considered to be very powerful and effective antibiotics, resistance is not unusual, as many bacteria develop methods of keeping the aminoglycosides from entering their cells in the first place, thereby making it impossible to block the formation of new protein.

When administered by injection, the aminoglycosides are distributed throughout the body's tissues, with the exception of the central nervous system. They are not effective in crossing the blood-brain barrier, even when these tissues are inflamed. The patient's body does not alter these antibiotics and they are excreted unchanged by the kidneys into the urine. When given by injection they can be used to treat most types of infections, including those of the bladder.

However, if antibiotics of this group are given orally, they are not well absorbed from the intestine. Rather, most remain within the gastrointestinal tract and the portion that is not used passes out in the stool. They are usually intended to treat bacterial intestinal infections and they can be quite effective because most disease-causing organisms in this area are Gram-negative.

The aminoglycosides are frequently used in topical preparations that are applied on the skin, eyes, and ears of dogs. They are very effective at controlling bacterial infections in these areas and are frequently combined with steroids or other antimicrobials.

The problem with the aminoglycosides that prevents their more widespread use is the serious side effects associated with their usage. When injected at excessive levels or for prolonged periods of time, they may severely damage kidney and inner ear tissues. Affected kidneys may temporarily lose their ability to eliminate wastes from the blood, and in some cases could fail completely. Animals with inner ear toxicity may lose the ability to maintain their balance and will walk with an abnormal gait. Some animals may also lose some degree of hearing. All of these abnormalities may return to normal after the medication is discontinued, but in some patients the loss will be permanent. Toxic side effects in the kidneys or the inner ear structures are much more likely to occur in animals that are concurrently being treated with a furosemide diuretic (Lasix).

Topical preparations may also lead to toxicity if significant quantities of the antibiotics enter deeper areas of the body. An example of this would be an ear preparation used when the eardrum has been ruptured or lanced, allowing easy access to the inner ear.

The Tetracycline Antibiotic Group

First isolated in the 1940s, this group of antibiotics continues to enjoy wide usage today. Medications commonly utilized are **tetracycline, chlortetracycline, oxytetracycline, doxycycline,** etc. Some are still isolated from natural cultures of other microorganisms, while most are at least partially formulated in the laboratory. They are prepared in topical, oral, and injectable forms for use against a wide range of microorganisms. They are bacteriostatic, i.e., only inhibiting the growth and development of the bacteria, therefore relying on the immune system of the patient to play some part in the actual elimination of the disease-causing organisms. They are considered broad spectrum, with both Gram-positive and Gram-negative antibacterial activity, and are effective against rickettsial, chlamydial, and mycoplasmal organisms. Additionally, as will be seen in later chapters, they are also used against several internal parasites of dogs.

The tetracycline antibiotics enter the bacterial cell and inhibit the organism's protein synthesis. Resistance of bacteria frequently develops against the tetracyclines and this is usually accomplished by preventing its entrance through the bacterial cell wall.

When taken orally or by injection, the tetracyclines are spread through most areas of the body via the bloodstream. These medications are able to pass across the blood-brain barrier and enter the central nervous system. The tetracyclines do have a unique feature in that they combine readily with calcium. This causes some problems in both absorption and distribution. *Milk and milk by-products are high in calcium, which often becomes attached to the tetracyclines, preventing their absorption in the gastrointestinal tract when administered orally.*

The portion of tetracyclines that are absorbed into the system are excreted either via the kidneys through the urine or to a lesser degree by the liver through bile, which is passed out with the stool.

The tetracyclines are used to treat an extremely wide range of microorganisms including numerous bacterial and single-celled parasite species. Today, doxycycline is one of the preferred treatments for Lyme disease, a bacterial disorder. In some oral preparations they are combined with other medications in the treatment of bacterial intestinal infections. They interact with few other medications, but some drugs, such as phenobarbital and Dilantin (which are used to control seizures in epileptics), affect their dosage levels. These medications stimulate the liver, which then breaks down the tetracyclines at faster than normal rates.

Additionally, there are numerous topical tetracycline preparations formulated to treat eye, ear, and skin infections. These may be combined with steroids or other antimicrobials.

Most problems associated with tetracycline therapy are related to the fact that it often binds with calcium and becomes a part of the teeth and bones. This can be a problem in puppies, as it can lead to discoloration of teeth if they are exposed to it while the dentine and enamel are forming. The tetracyclines make their way into the uterus and are also passed through the milk. For this reason, these antibiotics should not be used in pregnant or nursing females or puppies under one year of age. Additionally, after oral administration, some dogs also have brief problems with vomiting and diarrhea.

THE LINCOSAMIDE GROUP

The **lincosamide** group contains **lincomycin** (Lincocin) and **clindamycin** (Antirobe). They are bacteriostatic, affecting only Gram-positive bacteria. They are produced in both injectable and orally administered forms. They inhibit new protein formation by the bacterial organism.

When given orally, food present in the gastrointestinal tract may significantly decrease the quantity absorbed, and it is therefore recommended that these products be given on an empty stomach. When given by injection, they spread to most areas of the body, but do not pass into the central nervous system. As the medications flow through the liver they are altered but still retain their effectiveness. Excretion occurs both via the kidneys through the urine and by the liver through the bile and stool.

The lincosamides are used to treat Gram-positive infections of the bone and soft tissues. Many veterinarians frequently use them in the treatment of skin infections. Some mycoplasmal organisms can also be successfully treated with the lincosamides.

The lincosamides cause very few side effects in the dog, with the exception of occasional diarrhea and vomiting. Problem interactions with other medications are also quite rare.

THE MACROLIDE GROUP

Among those included in this group, **erythromycin, oleandomycin,** and **tylosin** (Tylan) are commonly used in canine medicine. All are considered bacteriostatic and generally are more effective against the Gram-positive bacteria than against the Gram-negative ones. Tylosin has nearly an equal effect on Gram-negative bacteria as well as other microorganisms such as mycoplasma, rickettsia, and chlamydia. As with many other bacteriostatic antibiotics, this group functions by inhibiting new protein formation. In most cases, they may require some participation by the patient's own immune system to eliminate the bacteria in question.

The macrolides come in oral and injectable forms. Once given, they spread throughout the patient's body. They rarely, if ever, cross into the central nervous system through the blood-brain barrier. The majority of these medications that enter the body are deactivated or altered by the liver and pass out through the bile-stool route. A small portion is eliminated through the urine, but not enough to make them a drug of choice in treating urinary tract infections. They are used in a wide form of infections caused by either bacterial, mycoplasmal, or chlamydial organisms. Historically, tylosin has frequently been used very successfully to treat, among other disorders, respiratory tract infections and chronic colitis.

The most consistent side effect seen with macrolide usage occurs when erythromycin is given orally. Many patients have difficulty with this antibiotic when it is given in this fashion; severe vomiting and diarrhea often occur. This can also occur with tylosin but much less frequently. With this exception, the macrolides cause very few side effects and are, in fact, considered some of the safest antibiotics for use in dogs. Additionally, they can be used synergistically with aminoglycosides such as gentamicin or some of the sulfonamides. However, they are definitely antagonistic with chloramphenicol and drugs of the lincosamide group.

Chloramphenicol

This bacteriostatic antibiotic is considered to have a broad spectrum of activity affecting both Gram-positive and Gram-negative organisms. It also has some effect against the mycoplasma and chlamydia disease-causing organisms although it is rarely used in these cases. It is found in oral and injectable forms as well as a wide range of topical preparations. It is usually sold generically under the name of **chloramphenicol** or referred to as **chloromycetin.** When given systemically, that is through oral or injectable routes, it spreads throughout the body. It reaches the structures of the central nervous system, easily passing through the blood-brain barrier, and has the potential to be used for a wide range of infections involving many different tissues of the body—but, as will be discussed, its popularity has fallen greatly.

Chloramphenicol is metabolized by the liver into forms that are generally inactive. Unlike many products that are broken down by the liver, this antibiotic is excreted via the kidneys and urine whether in its active or degraded form.

In canine medicine, especially in the oral and injectable forms, chloramphenicol usage has decreased greatly over the last two decades. Today the various potentially serious side effects of this medication are well understood! Many animals suffer from gastrointestinal upsets with diarrhea or vomiting while on the medication. In some cases, these can be severe.

More serious, however, is the potential for suppression of bone marrow function. Some individuals on this product will fail to release new red and white blood cells into circulation; there are instances in which treated patients will completely shut down production of these necessary cells. This can be fatal if the syndrome is not reversed, as a depressed number of red blood cells can lead to severe anemia. Remember, the red blood cells are responsible for carrying oxygen throughout the body. Additionally, animals with an insufficient quantity of white blood cells (the body's first line of defense against disease-causing microorganisms) may easily succumb to otherwise mild or non-disease-causing microoganisms. None of these problems occur with topical preparations and because of that, this antibiotic is still fairly popular in eye and ear ointments and solutions.

Bacitracin
This bactericidal antibiotic functions by destroying the cell wall of the microorganism. It is only effective against Gram-positive bacteria. Used in topical preparations it is quite safe but if given systematically, kidney damage can occur. Its use in canine medicine is generally restricted to topical lotions and ointments and in these preparations it is frequently combined with polymyxin B or neomycin.

Polymyxin B
This antibiotic is bactericidal, directly attacking the cell membranes of microorganisms. It is used predominantly against Gram-negative bacteria although it is also effective against some Gram-positive ones. In canine medicine, its use is generally restricted to topical preparations and it is very safe when used in this form. There are systemic forms but it has the potential for severe toxic side effects on the kidneys and various neural tissues.

In topical medications it has been found to work synergistically with bacitracin, neomycin, and members of the tetracycline group and is therefore frequently combined with them.

THE NON-ANTIBIOTIC ANTIBACTERIALS

These medications are not derived or designed from naturally occurring by-products of microorganisms as are antibiotics. Rather, they have been developed independently through research that tests the effect of chemicals on disease-causing microorganisms. They are then manufactured in the laboratory.

The Sulfonamides

The **sulfonamides** comprise a large and very useful group of medications. They are not antibiotics as they are not produced by microorganisms. Rather, they are manufactured in laboratories. They are exceptionally effective against many bacterial and other microorganismal species. Although their use dates back to the 1930s, they have continually been improved and updated and today are used routinely in canine medicine. They can be used by themselves, in combination therapy with other antibacterials, or to greatly increase their efficacy they may be formulated specifically together with one of the diaminopyrimidines (i.e., trimethoprim) or diaminobenzylpyrimidines (i.e., ormetoprim).

When used by themselves, the sulfonamides are bacteriostatic at normal concentrations or dosage levels, affecting new protein formation by microorganisms. Because of this, they are most efficient when the bacterial species being treated is in an acute or rapidly multiplying stage. They are not very effective in the treatment of chronic infections as these bacteria are more quiescent, with less new protein formation occurring. They are effective against Gram-positive and Gram-negative bacteria, chlamydia, and protozoan parasites such as toxoplasmosis and coccidiosis. Specific examples of sulfonamides in this group are **sulfanilamide, sulfamethazine, sulfadimethoxine** (Albon or Bactrovet), **sulfamerazine, sulfadiazine, sulfasalazine,** etc. Occasionally, members of this group are commercially formulated together and are more effective when used together than separately. An example of this would be the "Triple Sulfa" preparations or tablets that contain sulfamethazine, sulfamerazine, and sulfadiazine.

When given orally or by injection, these sulfas are distributed widely throughout the body with effective concentrations being attained in most tissues, including those of the central nervous system. The body works to break down or inactivate these medications by a variety of processes. They are finally excreted by the body through the kidneys and urine, although some is eliminated through the liver via the bile-stool pathway. Much of the product that is excreted through the urine is still in the active, pre-metabolized form and therefore the sulfonamides are used to treat kidney or bladder infections.

In the lactating dog, a portion is also excreted through the milk and this must be considered, as unwanted levels may be reached in nursing puppies. However, the sulfonamides are used to treat infections in all tissues of the body. There are variations in the absorption or distribution of different sulfas in this class and sometimes these differences can be used advantageously in treating different organisms or sites within the patient's body.

Resistance to the sulfonamides by microorganisms often develops during a course of therapy; if it is noted that the medication seems to be losing its effectiveness, a switch to a different medication must be made or another "culture and sensitivity" done.

A second and very important group of the sulfas are the "potentiated sulfonamides." The strengthening of these products is done by combining them with trimethoprim or ormetoprim. These combinations are bactericidal, being much more effective against both Gram-positive and Gram-negative bacterial populations regardless of whether they are in an acute or chronic phase. Specific examples would be **sulfadimethoxine-ormetoprim** (Primor), **sulfadiazine-trimethoprim** (Tribrissen), and numerous generic formulations. These are well absorbed throughout the body by oral administration or an injectable route. Almost all tissues are well profused with the active form of the products, including those of the central nervous system. Resistance does not occur as frequently or as rapidly with these combination products as it does when a sulfonamide is used by itself.

Unwanted side effects can and do occur with any of the sulfonamides whether they are of the "potentiated" variety or not. The **trimethoprim** or **ormetoprim** portion of the potentiated sulfas are very safe and cause few problems. However, the various sulfas all have the potential to cause kidney damage, especially in those animals with previously impaired kidney function or in those patients that have inadequate fluid levels or intake. The sulfonamides must be flushed through the kidneys to be cleared into the urine and this requires ample water. In dehydrated or stressed animals or those with less than normal levels of fluid intake, these medications build up within the kidneys, causing severe and even life-threatening kidney damage.

Some patients will also develop mild hypersensitivity or allergic reactions in the form of skin rashes and gastrointestinal disturbances such as vomiting and diarrhea. Additionally, some patients will develop "dry eye syndrome," or keratitis sicca, which is characterized by less than normal tear production. Long term use of the "potentiated" sulfas has been reported to suppress normal thyroid activity, even to the point of producing clinical hypothyroidism. In most cases except for those of an allergenic nature, these adverse reactions can be avoided by maintaining adequate hydration of the patient and limiting the time the animal is on the medication. It is usually recommended that at normal dosage level, the sulfonamides not be used for longer than seven to ten days and the "potentiated" ones be limited to ten to fourteen days.

The Quinolones

These synthetically produced substances are formed from various carboxylic acid molecules. They are bactericidal, damaging the DNA molecules and genetic materials of the bacteria, thereby killing them and/or preventing multiplication. In canine medicine, one of the most commonly used members in the quinolone group is **enrofloxacin** (Baytril). This is an excellent product and in the last few years it has grown significantly in popularity with many veterinarians. Another example of a quinolone would be **ciprofloxacin** (Cipro). These are very effective against many Gram-positive and Gram-negative bacteria and some mycoplasma species. They are formulated in injectable and oral forms. Regardless of how they are administered, they are distributed throughout the body to most tissues, including the mammary glands and uterus. For some reason, therapeutic levels are usually not attained within the central nervous system or the bones.

Different quinolones are metabolized to varying degrees by the body but this rarely affects their activity within the body. They are excreted by the kidneys into the urine. They are therefore useful for treating infections of the lower urinary tract.

These are generally considered to be very safe for use in dogs. One problem rarely encountered is cartilage damage. This is usually noted in rapidly growing adolescent dogs. It should therefore not be used in these animals or in pregnant or nursing females. These products rarely interact with other medications but are generally not used in combination with other antimicrobials.

Metronidazole

Metronidazole (Flagyl) is most commonly thought of as an antiprotozoal medication used to treat *Giardia*. In recent years it has been found that this medication is also very useful against bacterial infections, especially those occurring within the intestinal tract. It is bactericidal, affecting many Gram-negative bacteria as well as some Gram-positive forms. The exact mechanism of action that the product utilizes against these bacterial species is not well understood. In today's dog, the medication is often used quite successfully in nonspecific diarrheal disorders in which a definitive diagnosis cannot be made. After oral administration, a portion of the product is absorbed into the general circulation and is distributed throughout the body, including into the central nervous system. Metronidazole is therefore effective against many bacterial organisms found throughout the body.

Most of the product is excreted through the kidneys and urine. A small portion is metabolized by the liver but this is unimportant to the dosage schedule.

At typical dosages, few side effects are noted with metronidazole usage in the dog. There are reports of the medication affecting bone marrow production and release of new blood cells. Additionally, there are references in the veterinary literature of animals treated with metronidazole showing signs that would indicate the product can cause some damage or irritation to neural tissue. These affected animals may seem dizzy, stagger, have difficulty maintaining normal posture, and/or tilt their heads to one side or the other. In the authors' experience, we have not seen any of these problems in the animals we have treated with this medication. We have seen a few animals exhibit mild gastrointestinal upsets such as vomiting and diarrhea. Because of potential side effects on the unborn, the product should not be used in pregnant females.

SUMMARY

Except for heartworm preventatives, the *antimicrobials used against bacteria and other small organisms are probably the most frequently dispensed products in veterinary medicine.* They are exceptionally useful. Although side effects do occur, the gain from their usage far outweighs any problems encountered.

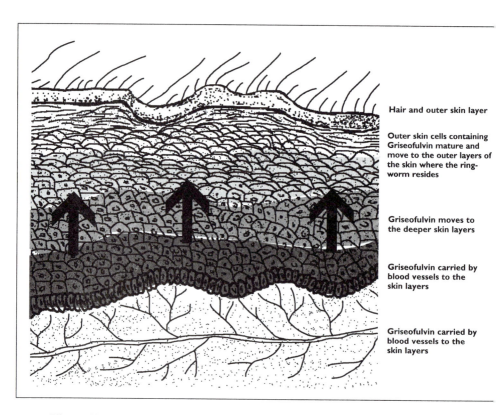

Hair and outer skin layer

Outer skin cells containing Griseofulvin mature and move to the outer layers of the skin where the ringworm resides

Griseofulvin moves to the deeper skin layers

Griseofulvin carried by blood vessels to the skin layers

Griseofulvin carried by blood vessels to the skin layers

Figure 5-1: Griseofulvin being carried through the skin as cells mature.

CHAPTER 5
Fungal and Yeast Infections

Fungal infections are fairly common in the dog. **Ringworm (dermatophytosis)** is the most frequently encountered and occurs throughout all areas of the United States. It is a skin disease that can have the typical isolated circular lesions. In other cases, large areas of the body may be involved. In the dog, it is usually caused by *Trichophyton* or *Microsporum* species. Collectively they are referred to as the **dermatophytes.**

Other fungal diseases, such as **blastomycosis, aspergillosis, coccidioidomycosis,** or **histoplasmosis,** etc., are caused by organisms of the same name but are usually more regional in location. Additionally, diseases such as **cryptococcus** or **candidiasis** are caused by yeasts of the same name. While ringworm, primarily a disease of the skin, is not usually considered a life-threatening disorder in dogs, many of the others mentioned above seriously affect internal body structures and often lead to death.

Griseofulvin

Griseofulvin (Fulvicin) has been used to treat dermatophytes for many years in this country. It is considered an antibiotic as it is produced by a microorganism, *Penicillium griseofulvin.* It has no effect on bacteria, but affects only fungal organisms, and only those that affect the skin and cause diseases such as ringworm. It has little or no effect on systemic fungal infections such as blastomycosis, histoplasmosis, coccidioidomycosis, etc.

It disrupts division and development of fungal organisms affecting the skin and is generally considered fungistatic. Griseofulvin is only administered orally. Unlike some medications, it should be taken with food, especially those with a high fat content as this improves its absorption by the gastrointestinal tract into the bloodstream. The product is deposited into the lower and most immature layers of the skin and must slowly be carried up through the skin as the various layers mature. (See Figure 5-1.) Because of this and its fungistatic action, therapy usually must be continued for several weeks or months to be effective.

In recent years, griseofulvin usage has been replaced by some of the newer medications, especially the azole derivatives. Most practitioners consider them to be more effective. Additionally, their action is much faster, allowing much shorter treatment schedules in cases of the dermatophytes. Most antifungal medications are expensive and shortened treatment time significantly decreases the overall cost of treatment for the client.

Griseofulvin is broken down by the liver and excreted through the kidneys. Serious side effects are rarely noted in treated animals although vomiting, diarrhea, and anemia may occur. When problems do occur with this product, it is generally in patients that suffer from some concurrent disease or dysfunction of the liver. These patients should be monitored closely when treated with this medication. *Griseofulvin can cause abnormalities in developing puppies within the uterus and should therefore not be given to pregnant females.*

AZOLE DERIVATIVES

This group contains **thiabendazole, miconazole** (Conofite), **clotrimazole** (Lotrimin), **econazole** (Ecostatin), **ketoconazole** (Nizoral), **fluconazole** (Diflucan), **itraconazole** (Sporanox), etc. The name of the active ingredient always has the "azole" suffix at the end of the word. They are formulated in topical, oral, and injectable preparations. In the last decade, their usage has increased greatly as veterinarians have found them to be very effective in treating superficial fungal infections of the skin such as ringworm as well as those affecting the various internal systems of the body. Prior to their development, many systemic infections could only be effectively treated with prolonged amphotericin B intravenous injections.

TOPICAL AZOLE DERIVATIVES

Miconazole, clotrimazole, thiabendazole, and econazole come in a wide range of topical preparations that are prescribed for everything from ringworm in animals to athlete's foot in people. Additionally, thiabendazole in topical preparations has been found to be effective against ear mites. In some of these products they are the only active ingredient, while in others they are mixed with different drugs to give the final preparation a broader spectrum. An example of this would be the topical solution Tresaderm that is frequently used in canine medicine for ear infections. It contains thiabendazole, dexamethasone (an anti-inflammatory steroid), and neomycin (an aminoglycoside antibiotic). Additionally, *there are numerous topical preparations containing these topical azole derivatives that are available in over-the-counter nonprescription forms.*

PARENTERALLY ADMINISTERED AZOLE DERIVATIVES

Ketoconazole, itraconazole, and **fluconazole** are the preferred medications today for systemic fungal infections. Prior to their development, only long term usage of amphotericin B injections were available for these infections (see page 49). Additionally, they may be used for some superficial infections. Of these newer medications, ketoconazole has been found to be very useful in the treatment of ringworm, often requiring a shorter course of treatment than would be necessary with griseofulvin. These medications are considered to be both fungistatic and fungicidal.

Ketoconazole is given orally in either tablet or liquid form. Dogs often exhibit gastrointestinal upsets such as vomiting, diarrhea, or loss of appetite when first on the medication. These problems can often be decreased or eliminated if the daily dosage is divided into two to three portions and given over the course of the day with food. In a very few animals, especially older ones or those with pre-existing liver problems, hepatotoxicity has been reported. In most animals, however, these signs disappear soon after the dosage is decreased or the medication is discontinued.

Ketoconazole also causes some unwanted effects on certain glandular structures. The medication may sometimes retard or eliminate sperm cell formation and lower blood levels of testosterone, the male hormone produced in the testicles. Additionally, it can also suppress the adrenal gland's production of hormones. Even treating hundreds and hundreds of cases of blastomycosis, we have had very few problems with this medication. As with griseofulvin, however, unless it is absolutely necessary, it should not be used in pregnant females as it may have detrimental effects on the unborn fetuses.

An interesting aspect of ketoconazole therapy is that it must be given for several days before it has a significant effect on fungal organisms. Therefore, when treating systemic fungal diseases, most clinicians prefer to treat the patient first with two to four intravenous injections of amphotericin B to rapidly arrest the growth and spread of the disease-causing organisms within the body. Ketoconazole works well with amphotericin B. Ketoconazole will often then be used for an additional 60 to 120 days in severe systemic fungal infections.

Most of the ketoconazole administered is broken down by the liver and excreted through the bile and into the stool. As stated, it is synergistic when used with amphotericin B. It should not be used together with griseofulvin as this greatly increases the potential for liver problems. Gastrointestinal antacids such as cimetidine or other over-the-counter drugs such as Tums or Rolaids should not be used while an animal is treated with ketoconazole as a more acid environment in the gut promotes absorption in the body.

While ketoconazole is still the most popular, fluconazole and itraconazole use has been increasing in the last few years. While they are not as effective against the dermatophytes that cause the superficial infections such as ringworm, these newer azole derivatives are equally effective against systemic fungal forms. Additionally, although they have the potential to produce the same side effects, these are usually milder than those observed with ketoconazole. The metabolism, distribution, and interactions with other drugs are identical to those of ketoconazole.

Flucytosine

Flucytosine (Ancobon) is usually thought of as an anticancer drug. It is given orally and readily absorbed from the gastrointestinal tract throughout the body. It even passes across the blood-brain barrier into the central nervous system. Flucytosine is considered fungistatic and works best when given concurrently with other antifungal products such as amphotericin B or ketoconazole. However, fungal organisms are reported to rapidly develop a resistance to flucytosine. This, combined with the fact that its spectrum of activity is not as broad as the azole derivatives, has caused some lack of popularity in canine medicine. Few side effects are noted except mild gastrointestinal upsets such as vomiting, diarrhea, or loss of appetite. It is almost totally excreted via the kidneys with little metabolism or alteration by the body.

Amphotericin B

This injectable product has become the workhorse in the early stages of treatment of many fungal diseases. This medication belongs to the macrolide antibiotic group. These are defined as antibiotics because they are produced by a microorganism, *Actinomyces*, and have inhibitory effects on other microbes. Depending on the concentration within the patient's body, amphotericin B can be either fungistatic or fungicidal. *It is a very caustic product* and must be given intravenously. Once administered, it is transported to most of the body but fails to reach significant or therapeutic levels within the central nervous system. The product is eliminated from the body unchanged through the urine or by breakdown in the liver. It is routinely used in conjunction with the azole derivatives with the mechanisms working together in synergistic fashion.

Amphotericin B, if not carefully monitored or if used for prolonged periods of time, can cause severe kidney toxicity, affecting the ability to eliminate toxic wastes from the body. In some cases these signs disappear after therapy is discontinued or with aggressive fluid therapy. In others, the effects on normal healthy tissue are too great and the patient may die.

Nystatin

Nystatin (Mycostatin) is closely related to amphotericin B but in canine medicine is only used topically. It is also considered an antibiotic, isolated from *Streptomyces* cultures. In these topical preparations it is considered fungistatic or fungicidal, depending on the concentration attained in the area of the disease-causing organism. It is usually effective against yeasts such as candida and various dermatophytes.

MISCELLANEOUS TOPICAL ANTIFUNGAL PREPARATIONS

There are miscellaneous solutions or creams that are manufactured and labeled for topical use against dermatophyte fungal organisms. These usually have sulfur, copper, or iodine compounds as their active ingredients. One example of a sulfur medication is LymDyp which can be used as a treatment for fleas and several types of mites.

Except in very minor cases or those having only extremely localized lesions, these preparations are usually used in conjunction with
azole derivatives or griseofulvin. In the authors' experience, if used
by themselves in minor cases these can be helpful in eliminating
topical fungal infections if treatment is initiated early in the course
of the disease. Examples of these products would be Fungisan, Betadine, etc.

CHAPTER 6

Medications Used Against Viruses

Medications, as we typically think of them, are rarely used against viral organisms in canine medicine. In most situations, the animal's immune system is responsible for developing an immunity and expelling the virus from the body. This kind of action is seen routinely in human diseases such as colds. In veterinary medicine, the defense against viral diseases is usually accomplished using vaccines in a preventative manner.

There *are* medications available for the treatment of viruses. All of these are human drugs that have occasionally been used in dogs. As would be expected, each has a specific spectrum of activity, being useful only against certain viral organisms. These may be administered topically, orally, or via injection. Among those that may be prescribed for oral use are **amantadine, ancyclovir** (Zovirax), and **ribavirin** (Virazole). Topical products include **vidarabine, trifluridine,** and **idoxuridine.**

All of these products are expensive and, with rare exceptions, can cause serious side effects. Viruses live within the cells of the host animal and use the cellular structures of the infected animal to reproduce. Most medications that affect viruses will therefore affect the host's normal cellular activity to some degree. Because of these factors, the short course of most viral diseases, and the inability to make a specific diagnosis within that time, these medications are rarely used and are beyond the scope of this book.

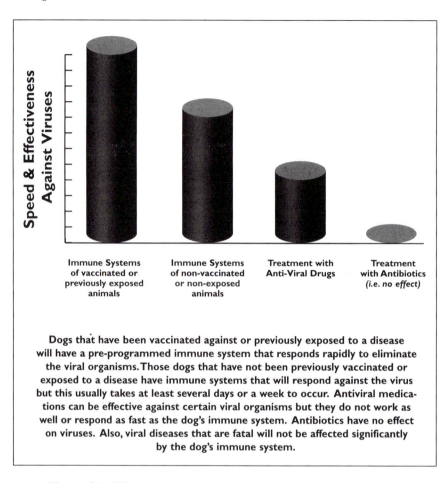

Dogs that have been vaccinated against or previously exposed to a disease will have a pre-programmed immune system that responds rapidly to eliminate the viral organisms. Those dogs that have not been previously vaccinated or exposed to a disease have immune systems that will respond against the virus but this usually takes at least several days or a week to occur. Antiviral medications can be effective against certain viral organisms but they do not work as well or respond as fast as the dog's immune system. Antibiotics have no effect on viruses. Also, viral diseases that are fatal will not be affected significantly by the dog's immune system.

Figure 6-1: Effectiveness against viruses by various treatments.

C H A P T E R   7

Medications for the Treatment of Internal Parasites

A parasite is an organism that lives in or on another animal. This means that the parasite lives and derives either nourishment and/or shelter from a host. In doing this, the parasite harms or steals nutrition from the other animal. In some cases, this can even lead to the death of the host.

Dogs have a wide range of internal parasites inside their bodies. The most common of these spend most of their lives in the gastrointestinal tract. Some steal from the food that the animal has eaten while others suck the host's blood through the wall of the intestine. Those most frequently encountered are **roundworms, hookworms, whipworms, tapeworms, coccidia,** and **giardia.**

Dirofilaria immitis, canine **heartworm,** spends its adult life within the dog's heart and large blood vessels of the lungs, damaging these structures and drawing nutrition from the blood. Figures 7-1 and 7-2 show the life cycles of the canine roundworm and heartworm as examples of those infecting dogs. **Roundworms, hookworms, whipworms,** and **heartworms** all belong to a larger group called nematodes. **Tapeworms** belong to the cestodes, and **coccidia** and **giardia** belong to the protozoans.

Most medications used against internal parasitic infections are designed to eliminate a current problem. All of the dog's parasites have complicated life cycles with the organism and develop through several different larval and adult forms. Some antiparasitic medications eliminate only certain stages of the parasites. Most of these preparations are only able to deal with the parasites while they are residing in certain areas of the dog's body. It is important that this

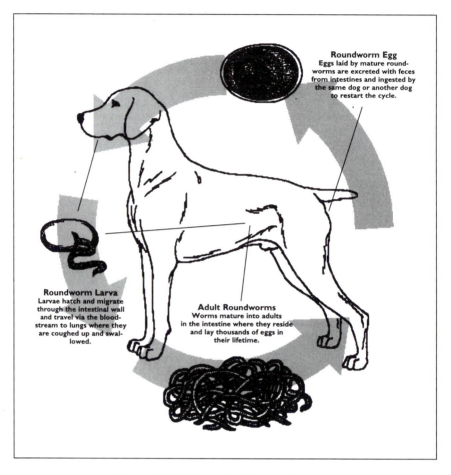

Roundworm Egg
Eggs laid by mature roundworms are excreted with feces
from intestines and ingested by
the same dog or another dog
to restart the cycle.

Roundworm Larva
Larvae hatch and migrate
through the intestinal wall
and travel via the blood-
stream to lungs where they
are coughed up and swal-
lowed.

Adult Roundworms
Worms mature into adults
in the intestine where they reside
and lay thousands of eggs in
their lifetime.

Figure 7-1: Life cycle of a roundworm.

limitation be understood, as during their life cycle most parasites
reside or migrate through several areas of the host's body. For most
parasites that live as adults in the dog's intestine, the medications
used to eliminate them only function on those forms that are in the
gastrointestinal tract.

When antiparasitic drugs are described as "preventative," this
is, in the strict sense of the word, not true. These drugs do not prevent them but rather allow the dog to become infected and then eliminate the parasite in a very early stage of the disease. For example,

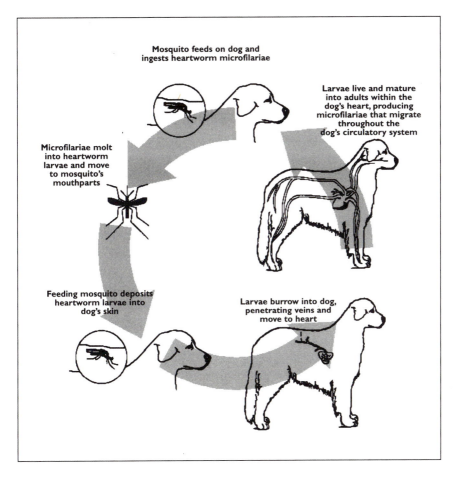

Figure 7-2: Heartworm life cycle.

heartworm pills are given on a monthly basis as a "preventative." As shown in Figure 7-2, a mosquito transmits the heartworm larvae through its bite. At that point in time, the dog has a living parasite drawing nourishment, causing tissue damage, and finding a space to live at the expense of the host. An ivermectin product (e.g., Heartgard-30) will kill the larval heartworm before it reaches the heart. Preventative antiparasitic drugs usually indicate that the organism is eliminated before it reaches the adult and most damaging form.

While most of these products do an excellent job of preventing the destructive stage of these internal parasites, it is not always possible, practical, or safe to be constantly giving a parasiticide. Additional measures must be taken to truly protect the dog. **Round-worm** and **whipworm** infections in adult dogs come from eating or licking something that has been contaminated by the stools of another already infected animal. **Hookworm** eggs pass out in the stool of the infected dog, hatch, and burrow through the skin or pads of another dog, entering its body. **Tapeworm** eggs also pass out with the stool, but these are not effective against another dog. Rather, these eggs are eaten by fleas, beetles, mice, or rabbits, which are referred to as "intermediate hosts." They are then eaten by another dog and *this* animal becomes infected, with an adult tapeworm developing in its intestines. With any of these parasites, the owner should do all that is possible to prevent the animal from coming in contact with the sources of the infection. Not using public areas to walk the pet, eliminating intermediate hosts such as fleas, not letting their dogs eat dead rabbits or mice, and using sprays to repel mosquitoes are good common sense measures to help prevent parasitic infections.

PROTOZOAN PARASITES

The protozoa are microscopic, single-celled animals. A few of these are parasites of dogs. Their treatment often utilizes antibiotics or other antimicrobials that are most commonly used against bacteria. Generally speaking, these medications are more effective against bacteria than they are when used against these single-celled parasites. Sulfadimethoxine, metronidazole, and the tetracyclines are all prescription products.

Sulfadimethoxine
Sulfadimethoxine is one of the sulfonamide antimicrobials frequently used to treat bacterial infections. It is also the preferred medication used to control the gastrointestinal parasitic disease **coccidiosis,** and is available in injectable and oral forms. It is sold as a generic or under the brand names Albon or Bactrovet. Sulfadimethoxine is unique as an antiparasitic drug in that it does not kill the parasite but only inhibits its growth. It is therefore said to be coccidiostatic. Animals treated for coccidiosis with this drug are

usually on the medication for ten to twelve days. For a more complete discussion of the properties of the sulfonamides, please see chapter 4.

Metronidazole

Metronidazole (Flagyl) is a member of the nitroimidazole group of antimicrobials and is routinely used for the treatment of gastrointestinal disorders, often when no definitive diagnosis can be made. Additionally, it is the preferred medication used to treat *giardia* species infections. This single-celled parasite lives in the intestinal tract of dogs. They usually acquire the infection by drinking fecally contaminated water. A discussion of metronidazole can be found in chapter 4.

TETRACYCLINE ANTIMICROBIALS

This group of antibiotics is used to treat most of the **rickettsial parasites** including *Ehrlichia, Rickettsia,* and *Neorickettsia* species that are responsible for such diseases as Rocky Mountain spotted fever, Salmonella poisoning, and infectious thrombocytopenia and ehrlichiosis.

Of the tetracyclines, those most commonly used to treat these diseases are **oxytetracycline, tetracycline,** and **doxycycline.** When treating bacterial diseases with these products, the duration of treatment is usually less than fourteen days. However, with parasitic infections, the medications take longer to be effective and relapses are common. Treatment is therefore often extended for a period of several weeks or months. Longer usage increases the potential for the side effects associated with the tetracyclines, such as gastrointestinal upsets like vomiting or diarrhea, discoloration of developing teeth, etc. For a more complete discussion of the tetracyclines, see chapter 4.

WORMS (GASTROINTESTINAL)

While the roundworms, hookworms, whipworms, and tapeworms sometimes seem to have little in common except that they all reside as adults in the intestinal tract of the dog, their similarities often allow them to be treated with the same medication.

The worming medications of today are much safer and easier on the patient than those popular only a decade ago. Serious adverse reactions are quite rare with the newer antiparasitic drugs. Most of today's products can be given with or without food, on a full or empty stomach, rarely cause diarrhea or vomiting, and animals living in areas where parasite numbers are very high can be safely treated on a frequent basis. Some can be used on puppies as young as two weeks of age and others given to pregnant bitches.

Most importantly, the drugs we use against gastrointestinal parasites today are very effective. In a single administration, they typically eliminate 85 to 98 percent of the worms present. Unfortnately, they only kill or affect the parasites located within the intestines.

Many of the worms found in the gut have larval forms in other tissues of the body. Hookworm and roundworm larvae can be found in the lungs, uterus, and mammary glands; wormers have no effect on these forms. Some of these products kill the adult parasites while others only paralyze them so that they are carried from the body normally.

Piperazine

This is one of the oldest wormers still in use today. It is available in many over-the-counter formulations that can be purchased without a prescription. While it has some effect on other parasites, it is considered effective only in the removal of roundworms. The only consistent side effect is vomiting. If this occurs, it will usually be within the first hour after administration. Piperazine paralyzes the parasite and carries it out through the gastrointestinal tract. In very rare instances, as when excessively high dosages have been accidentally given, signs associated with the nervous system are observed. This can vary from a mild body shaking to seizures.

Piperazine is given orally and is available in liquid, tablets, or capsules, and is commonly sold over-the-counter without a prescription. Piperazine is commonly used in adults and puppies over six weeks of age. The worming is usually repeated in two and four weeks. This allows the forms of the parasite that are migrating through the dog's body to reach the intestine where the medication is effective.

Pyrantel Pamoate

This wormer for dogs is usually sold under the brand names of Nemex, Nemex 2, and Evict. It is also formulated for horses in a more concentrated form sold under the name Strongid T. It is also a component in Heartgard-30 Plus. Most forms labeled for dogs are available over-the-counter without a prescription. Pyrantel pamoate is orally administered and manufactured in liquid and tablet forms. It is not absorbed from the intestines very well, which allows it to remain in the gut where its activity is needed. This also decreases the possibility of side effects. Pyrantel is a **cholinesterase inhibitor,** which is discussed in chapter 8, on the ectoparasites. Most drugs in this class have the potential to cause severe adverse reactions. But since pyrantel pamoate is not absorbed into the bloodstream of the dog, these problems are avoided.

In cases in which roundworms and/or hookworms are the only parasites present or to be prevented, this is without a doubt the most popular canine wormer with veterinarians and breeders today. It is incredibly safe and effective. Puppies can be wormed as early as two weeks of age. It eliminates over 90 percent of the hookworms and roundworms present with a single treatment. The only adverse sign noted is vomiting within the first hour after administration and this is very rare. It is believed that this is caused by the increased movement of the parasites as they react to the pyrantel pamoate.

With this product, it is recommended that puppies be wormed at two, three, five, and seven weeks of age. The mother should also be wormed at the same time. Remember that roundworms and hookworms lodge in the uterus and mammary glands, passing on to the puppies during pregnancy and lactation. Early worming is done with this product to eliminate them before they become a significant problem in the pups. The mother is wormed because she usually cleans and ingests the stools of the newborn, thereby reinfecting herself. Pyrantel pamoate is not able to kill the parasites that reside in the uterus or mammary glands. In most cases, the puppies will already have roundworms and hookworms in these tissues before or soon after birth, creating a source of parasitism for their future litters.

Adults, except nursing mothers, are usually wormed two or three times in succession, with each treatment being separated by two weeks. Roundworms and hookworms migrate through the body before reaching the intestines. Pyrantel pamoate is only effective against them after they reach that area of the body. Treatments are therefore repeated to coincide with their approximate arrival in the intestines.

Toluene

This is one of the older wormers and can be purchased without a prescription. Toluene is one of the active ingredients found in the "triple wormer capsules" sold under such brand names as Trivermicide. Because of its taste and irritating properties to the mouth, it is usually formulated in large gelatin capsules.

This is one of the few antiparasitic products used against the large parasites of the gut today that requires that food be withheld for twelve hours prior to administration and for an additional four hours afterward. It has relatively good activity against roundworms and hookworms but is not as safe or effective as pyrantel pamoate. An additional problem with toluene is that it is packaged in such large capsules, which are very difficult to administer. The product is not usually used in puppies younger than seven weeks of age.

Dichlorvos

This organophosphate is sold under the brand name Task for dogs. It is a prescription product. Administered orally, it is available in tablets or granules that can be mixed with food. It is effective against roundworms, hookworms, and whipworms but only when they are in the intestinal tract. Organophosphates are cholinesterase inhibitors and the problems with their usage are discussed in chapter 8, on ectoparasites. In the last few years, the popularity and usage of this product has decreased greatly. An additional problem with Task is that it can never be used in a dog with canine heartworm disease. *It kills all of the heartworms at once, causing a anaphylactic reaction that may lead to the death of the dog.*

Mebendazole

Mebendazole, sold under the name Telmintic, is produced in a powder form that is to be added to food. It is a prescription product and is effective against roundworms, hookworms, whipworms, and certain tapeworms. As with other gastrointestinal tract wormers, it has little or no effect on the migrating forms that are located in other parts of the body. Additionally, it is only effective against the *Taenia* species tapeworms that dogs contract when eating rabbits or mice. It has no effectiveness against the *Dipylidium* species tapeworms that are contracted from fleas. There have been reports of liver toxicity with this product and it should not be used in a dog with any pre-existing liver disease. The popularity and usage of this product has decreased in the last few years. Other products have taken its place because of their wider margin of safety and effectiveness.

Fenbendazole

Fenbendazole has become one of the more popular canine wormers today. It is a prescription product and is sold under the brand name Panacur in a granular form that is mixed with food. There are also types formulated and labeled for horses. It is very effective against roundworms, hookworms, and whipworms. Additionally, it is also a preferred medication in the treatment of the *Taenia* species tapeworms which dogs contract by eating contaminated rabbits and mice. It has no effect against the *Dipylidium* species tapeworms that dogs get from eating fleas. At the typical dosages listed on the label, *Panacur is only effective against the above parasites when they are in the intestines.* However, it has been shown experimentally that if it is used for prolonged periods of time during pregnancy and lactation at elevated dosages, the roundworm and hookworm numbers in the newborn puppies are significantly reduced.

Fenbendazole is mixed with the dog's food for three consecutive days. This should be repeated in two to three weeks. The only side effects that are common with fenbendazole are vomiting in the first two hours after administration. Liver toxicity is not considered a problem, as is reported with mebendazole.

Dichlorophene

Dichlorophene is used against tapeworms. It is found in tablet form in such products as Happy Jack TapeWorm Tablets and is also formulated together with toluene in "triple wormer capsules," such as Happy Jack Trivermicide. All of these products are available as over-the-counter formulations and may therefore be purchased without a prescription. Even though this is a nonprescription product, it is highly effective in the removal of tapeworms with a single worming. It eliminates over 70 percent of all *Taenia* species infestations and approximately 85 percent of the *Dipylidium* species. If the treatment is repeated in two to three weeks, most problems are eliminated if there is no reinfestation.

Food should be withheld for twelve hours before and four hours *after* administration. Some vomiting and diarrhea is common in the first twelve hours after treatment. When given in the "triple wormer capsule" form that is combined with the active ingredient toluene, administration is often difficult. These capsules are very large when compared to the size of dog for which they are manufactured.

Praziquantel

Praziquantel is a prescription product sold under the name Droncit. It is very effective against both *Taenia* and *Dipylidium* species tapeworms. It is formulated in tablets that may be given with or without food, on a full or empty stomach. Injectable forms are also on the market. The medication destroys the coating that protects the parasite against the digestive juices of the dog. The tapeworm then dies and is often digested as raw protein by the dog. Sometimes little or no evidence of the parasite may be seen in the stool after treatment. Most veterinarians recommend that the treatment be repeated in two to three weeks.

The medication is swallowed, absorbed by the intestinal wall, and carried by the blood system to the liver where it is metabolized into the active form. It is then excreted in the bile back into the intestine in the active antiparasitic form.

Dogs treated with Droncit will occasionally vomit or have mild diarrhea following treatment, but other more serious signs are rarely if ever noted. This is an extremely safe and effective product. It can be used in puppies as young as four weeks of age. It can also be used in pregnant animals. There are no listed contraindications for its usage in adult dogs.

Epsiprantel

This tapewormer is sold under the brand name Cestex in tablets that can be given with or without food on a full or empty stomach. It is very safe and effective. In only rare instances will dogs vomit after it has been administered. It eliminates the parasite's protection from the dog's digestive juices. The body of the treated tapeworm may be digested and absorbed by the dog. Therefore, there may be little or no evidence of the infestation in the stool of the dog following treatment.

After oral administration, the medication is carried to the intestinal tract. It is not absorbed or altered by the body, but works immediately on any tapeworms present.

It can be used on puppies as young as seven weeks of age but is not cleared for use in pregnant animals. It is not known to interact with any other medications nor is it contraindicated in dogs with pre-existing medical conditions.

IVERMECTINS

This group of medications made their way into canine medicine in the 1980s. Since that time they have grown immensely in popularity and usage. They were originally only used as heartworm preventatives. Now some of these products are labeled to prevent other parasites; however, veterinarians frequently use these products in the treatment of numerous other parasitic problems for which they are not yet labeled or approved. The two products labeled for use in dogs are **ivermectin** (Heartgard-30) and **milbemycin oxime** (Interceptor). These are both prescription "once-a-month" medications used for heartworm prevention.

Ivermectin in this formulation kills the larval heartworms after they get into the dog's body. This happens before they reach the heart and blood vessels of the lungs. Heartgard-30 can be purchased in tablet or chewable treat form. It can also be purchased as a chewable treat that has pyrantel pamoate incorporated into the formulation (Heartgard-30 Plus) so that it also eliminates roundworm and hookworm infestations on a monthly basis. Animals as young as six weeks of age can be placed on these preparations. Animals usually remain on the product for life. It is used through pregnancy, lactation, and most illnesses.

Dogs should be tested to ensure that they are free of a pre-existing infestation of adult heartworms and/or microfilariae before treatment with ivermectin is initiated. Those infected should be treated to remove all adult and circulating microfilariae and only then can these animals be placed on any of the Heartgard-30 products. Severe hypersensitivity reactions can occur in animals with circulating microfilariae, which the medication can kill immediately.

Once on the medication, most practitioners still recommend that the dog be tested at least yearly for heartworm even if the animal remains on the product.

Collies are more sensitive to the ivermectin products. In this breed, the medication has the ability to cross the blood-brain barrier more easily and reach high concentrations within the brain. This can lead to toxic problems, with signs varying from staggering and loss of balance to seizures, coma, and death. It should be noted, however, that these signs are generally only seen when individuals use other ivermectin products at dosages much, much higher than those found in any of the Heartgard-30 products. The authors have treated numerous Collies with Heartgard-30 products without any problems being observed. It is still recommended that Collie owners closely observe their pets for the first eight to twelve hours following the initial administration.

Ivermectin products have come to be used for many things for which they are not yet labeled or approved. Ivomec, an injectable cattle wormer, is frequently used to treat a wide range of parasitic diseases in dogs. This nonprescription product has the same active ingredient as Heartgard-30. Veterinarians and breeders frequently use the solution in the treatment of sarcoptic mange, ear mites, nasal mites, and as an aid in the treatment of demodectic mange. Additionally, many breeders also use it in place of Heartgard-30 as a monthly heartworm preventative. Some choose to use it at elevated doses that are reported to eliminate infestations of roundworms, hookworms, and whipworms. There are other ivermectin products formulated for other large animals such as horses or pigs that are used in similar fashion by dog owners. Dog owners must understand that although these products may be very effective, they use them at their own risk. In the event that adverse reactions should occur, the manufacturer is in no way liable if products are used in ways for which they are not appropriately labeled.

Milbemycin oxime (Interceptor) also kills the heartworm larvae after they have entered into the dog's body. This occurs before they have reached the heart or blood vessels of the lungs. However, this product does have certain advantages over Heartgard-30. It also eliminates adult roundworm, hookworm, and whipworm infestations. Additionally, there are no labeled problems associated with its use in any breed. Puppies are placed on the medication as early as eight weeks of age. Dogs, including females that are pregnant and nursing can remain on the medication for life.

As with all heartworm products, it is important that adult dogs placed on milbemycin oxime first be blood tested to ensure that they are not already infested with adult and microfilarial forms of heartworm disease. If an animal already has the disease and is treated with Interceptor, the medication will probably kill large numbers of the microfilariae immediately, potentially leading to a fatal hypersensitivity reaction in the dog.

Diethylcarbamazine

This ingredient is found in several daily administered heartworm preventatives. Examples are Filaribits, Carbam, and Decacide. All of these are sold by prescription only. Filaribits are a chewable treat while Decacide and Carbam come in tablet, chewable tablet, or liquid form. While most animals will readily eat the chewable forms, the tablet and liquid styles are notorious for their bad taste. Some tablets are therefore coated.

Diethylcarbamazine kills the larval form of the heartworm parasite after it has entered the dog but before it has reached the heart or large blood vessels of the lungs. When administered in this fashion, it also aids in the prevention of roundworm infestations. Puppies are placed on diethylcarbamazine at two months of age. Dogs can be maintained on the product for life, including during pregnancy or while nursing. When an adult dog is being treated the first time with this medication, it should first have a blood test to ensure that it is not already infested with adult and microfilaria heartworms. *Treatment with this medication in an animal already harboring the parasite could easily lead to death as the adult heartworms would rapidly die and possibly clog the large blood vessels within the lungs.*

Diethylcarbamazine can also be used as a treatment of roundworm infestations but this is rarely done. Today, there are several products that are milder on the dog and more effective. It does not kill roundworms unless they are within the intestine. Treatment must therefore be repeated in two to three weeks, allowing those worms migrating through other tissues of the body to reach the gut so they may come in contact with the drug.

Some animals vomit soon after administration but this can usually be prevented if the products are given with food or soon after a meal.

Oxibendazole

This medication is formulated together with diethylcarbamazine in the prescription product Filaribits Plus. Its addition allows this daily administered product to also eliminate and prevent hookworm infestation and to be more effective in the elimination and prevention of roundworms.

Some problems with hepatotoxicity have been associated with Filaribits Plus usage that are not noted with regular Filaribits. This is thought to be due to the oxibendazole. It is relatively rare and signs are usually reversed when the medication is discontinued.

Owners should closely observe their animals for any abnormalities when they are first placed on this product. Additionally, the medication should not be used on dogs with a history of liver disease.

There are other internal parasites of the dog, but the ones listed comprise over 99 percent of infestations. Some of these additional forms require different medications than listed, but because of their rarity, they are considered outside of the scope of this book.

USING LARGE ANIMAL WORMERS IN DOGS

The term "large animal" here refers to farm animals such as cattle, horses, and pigs. In the above discussion on ivermectins it was mentioned that worming products formulated and labeled for large animals can be used in dogs. It is common today for veterinarians, breeders, and dog owners to choose these products for use in dogs. They have the same active ingredient and are made by the same manufacturer as those labeled for dogs. They are often much less expensive and can usually be purchased without a prescription in over-the-counter forms. We have rarely seen problems occur with this practice.

Individuals have the right to do this as long as they understand the risks. While they may be able to convert the large animal product to the exact same dog dosage, if anything goes wrong they themselves are completely responsible. The manufacturers of medical products have no liability if their products are used differently than described on the label. A wormer that states "For Use in Horses Only" on the label means that it has been formulated for and tested in horses. No claim is made about how the product will function in a dog or what adverse reactions might occur. If individuals choose to use these products on their own dogs, they should simply understand that they are responsible for any problems that might occur.

CHAPTER 8

The Treatment of Ectoparasites

A parasite is an organism that lives in or on another animal at whose expense it gains some benefit. The words "at whose expense" are important in differentiating parasites from other organisms that live together in a way that is beneficial to both parties. *Parasites always do some harm to, and may even kill, the hosts they live on or in.*

Specifically, the parasites that live on the surface of or within an animal's skin or body are called **ectoparasites.** In dogs, this includes **fleas, ticks, mites, lice,** and **biting flies.** Fleas, lice, and flies are insects with six legs while ticks and mites are arachnids (like spiders) that have eight legs. Insects and arachnids both belong to a larger group referred to as arthropods. Some of these parasites remain on the pet's body their entire lives while others may spend a portion living free in the environment. Sooner or later, however, they all attach themselves to the dog to feed. With most of these parasites, this means ingesting the blood, cells, or other material produced by the dog's body. A brief description of the parasites and their life cycles is included to better understand how the medications are used to eliminate or prevent these unwanted guests.

Of all the ectoparasites that affect dogs, **fleas** are the most common. They are typically only a seasonal problem in the northern United States, being dormant during the colder winter temperatures. In the South, however, they are a year-round nuisance. Figure 8-1 illustrates the life cycle of the common flea that infests dogs. The adult male and female fleas spend the majority of their lives on the dog's body. There they mate, with the female laying twenty to sixty eggs per day. These fall from the dog into the surrounding area and later hatch into free living larvae in the home or yard.

67

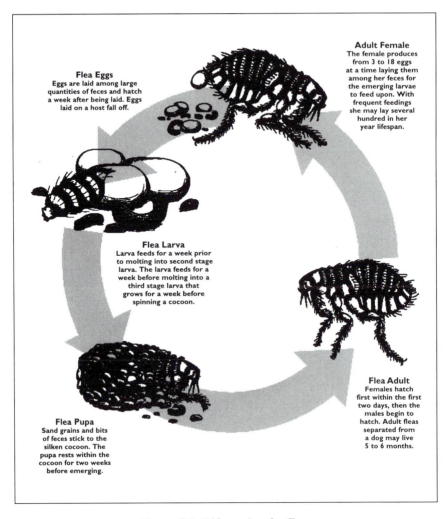

Adult Female
The female produces from 3 to 18 eggs at a time laying them among her feces for the emerging larvae to feed upon. With frequent feedings she may lay several hundred in her year lifespan.

Flea Eggs
Eggs are laid among large quantities of feces and hatch a week after being laid. Eggs laid on a host fall off.

Flea Larva
Larva feeds for a week prior to molting into second stage larva. The larva feeds for a week before molting into a third stage larva that grows for a week before spinning a cocoon.

Flea Pupa
Sand grains and bits of feces stick to the silken cocoon. The pupa rests within the cocoon for two weeks before emerging.

Flea Adult
Females hatch first within the first two days, then the males begin to hatch. Adult fleas separated from a dog may live 5 to 6 months.

Figure 8-1: Life cycle of a flea.

A developing flea goes through three different larval stages before transforming into a pupa within a cocoon. From this form an adult flea emerges, immediately seeking out a suitable host to feed on for the remainder of its life. Adults do jump off and on the dog or to other animals and humans.

Fleas are cold-blooded insects. Their life cycle is therefore affected by environmental temperature and humidity. Under perfect conditions, the entire life cycle from egg to adult can take as little as twelve days. In dry, cold conditions this process can take six months to complete. On average, from one generation to the next is a brief three to four weeks! In a single season, one female can be responsible for several hundred thousand descendants! The majority of fleas are not on the animal but living freely somewhere within the environment.

Therefore, to be effective, a majority of the efforts in the control or elimination of a flea problem must be aimed at the surroundings and not the pet. It is better to eliminate these parasites while they are in immature forms which do no harm to the pet, rather than wait for them to become adults that actively seek out dogs to parasitize.

Ticks are the second most common ectoparasite found on dogs. As with fleas, the adults feed on the dog, drawing blood directly through the skin of the pet. Their life cycle is different from fleas in that both adults and immature stages may feed on the dog. The stage of parasites coming in contact with the dog is important to remember when medications are used to either eliminate or prevent infestation.

At one time or another, everyone has found a large swollen tick somewhere on their dog, usually on or near the dog's head. The fur between the toes is also a common site, but in all honesty ticks can be anywhere on the animal. The immediate impression is that the tick is "engorged with blood." However, this enlarged tick is not filled with blood—it is filled with 2,000 to 8,000 eggs! The huge, swollen ticks that you find attached to your pet or crawling away from it are pregnant females. The eggs develop in the body of the female. She may expel them on the dog's body or drop off and deposit them within the home, kennel, or yard. Depending on the temperature and humidity, these hatch into larvae in two to eight weeks. They feed either on dogs or on some other kind of mammal. After a period of time, they molt into the next life stage of the tick, referred to as a nymph. The nymph feeds on the blood of a mammal just like the adult. After a varied period of time, nymphs mature into adults, thus completing the life cycle of the tick. See Figure 8-2.

Ticks are not fragile parasites. Under a wide variety of conditions, an individual adult can live for almost two years. Only very dry or very cold conditions have a serious adverse effect on these parasites. They love moist, warm weather. Typically, they are much more resistant to insecticidal products than are fleas.

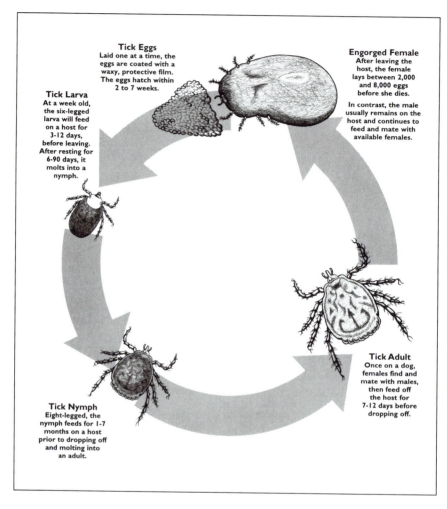

Tick Eggs
Laid one at a time, the eggs are coated with a waxy, protective film. The eggs hatch within 2 to 7 weeks.

Engorged Female
After leaving the host, the female lays between 2,000 and 8,000 eggs before she dies.

In contrast, the male usually remains on the host and continues to feed and mate with available females.

Tick Larva
At a week old, the six-legged larva will feed on a host for 3-12 days, before leaving. After resting for 6-90 days, it molts into a nymph.

Tick Adult
Once on a dog, females find and mate with males, then feed off the host for 7-12 days before dropping off.

Tick Nymph
Eight-legged, the nymph feeds for 1-7 months on a host prior to dropping off and molting into an adult.

Figure 8-2: Typical life cycle of a tick.

Mites, like ticks, are arachnids, responsible for "**mange.**" While some people confuse mange with many other disorders affecting the skin, the term correctly refers specifically to an infestation of mites. These organisms spend the majority of their lives on or under the surface of the dog's skin. Some mites live beneath the surface in tunnels they make, traversing back and forth through the deeper layers of the skin (e.g., *Sarcoptes scabiei*, which is responsible for scabies) or deep within hair follicles (e.g., *Demodex canis*, which causes demodicosis or "red mange"). Surface dwellers are the ear mite (*Otodectes cynotis*) and *Cheyletiella* which causes a generalized skin condition referred to as "walking dandruff." As would be expected, those that live on the surface of the animal's body are much easier to eliminate than those residing deeper within the skin.

The life cycle of mites can be considered in much simpler terms. They do pass through the same stages as ticks, i.e., adult, egg, larva, nymph, and back to adult again. However, all stages of the mite remain and feed on the dog. They quickly perish when off their host. With only a few exceptions, transmission to another dog usually occurs when these animals come in direct contact with each other. Treatment of the environment is therefore not as important as in cases involving fleas or ticks where the various life stages can exist for long periods off the host.

Today, infestations of dog **lice** are fairly uncommon in most areas of the United States. Other species of this group of insects commonly infest farm animals, birds, and occasionally children. Louse infestations of any animal are referred to as **pediculosis** and are typically very easy to treat, as the parasites spend their entire life cycle on the surface of the host's skin. They either draw blood from the host or live off its skin and hair.

Flies and **mosquitoes** rarely pose a severe threat to dogs. Under some circumstances, when animals are soiled with organic matter, flies may lay their eggs in the soiled areas, resulting in severe irritation caused by their larvae (i.e., maggots). In the summer or the Southern climates, certain biting varieties are also capable of causing irritation to the face and ears. Flies and mosquitoes also pose some threat in that they can be vectors or carriers of more serious diseases (e.g., heartworms).

TREATMENT PRINCIPLES

Treatment of an ectoparasitic problem, or preventing one from occurring, involves the use of a wide range of products combined with a good knowledge of the parasite's life cycle. If the target organism lives entirely on the host, then the treatment need only be directed there. If the parasite lives equally well off the dog as in the case of fleas and ticks, that portion of the population must also be considered. Usually this involves some application of insecticidal products in the general environment of the dog.

This is not true of mites and lice as they have great difficulty existing away from the dog's body. In fact, they soon die if they fall from the animal. With these parasites, all treatment measures are directed at the host. As would be expected, mite or louse infestations are much easier to deal with and eliminate than those caused by fleas or ticks.

Several different products may be utilized at the same time. For example, if a house dog develops a flea infestation, it would be correct to first shampoo the animal and then dip it with an insecticidal product. At the same time, the home should be treated with sprays and foggers while the yard is being sprayed.

TREATMENT METHODS

We will soon deal with the individual ingredients found in the various products used to deal with ectoparasites. First, however, let us take a few moments and examine the methods by which they are applied or utilized.

Most active ingredients are formulated in a wide variety of preparations. **Pyrethrins** are one of the most common groups of flea and tick products used today, and can be found in shampoos, sprays to be used on the pet, sprays used in the home, sprays used in the yard, powders, foggers, etc. Therefore, even if you have a preference of active ingredients in one of these antiectoparasitic products, you still have a wide range of choices as to how you will apply it.

Prior to dipping, bathing, or using sprays near the face, it is recommended that some form of sterile ophthalmic ointment be placed in the eyes to prevent irritation or inflammation.

SHAMPOOS   There are literally hundreds of shampoos labeled for use against fleas, ticks, lice, and/or certain mites, with a wide range of active ingredients. They are very useful in helping to protect the pet from getting fleas, or in eliminating a current problem. However, they are rarely adequate by themselves in controlling or preventing a problem. Since the lather produced by a shampoo is usually rinsed from the coat to prevent excessive drying of the skin and hair, much of the insecticidal properties are also removed from the animal. Insecticidal shampoos should be used with the idea that they will cleanse the coat, kill most of the parasites that are on the pet at that time, and hopefully leave some residual activity on the animal. To get the maximum effect from a shampoo, the animal should be allowed to "drip dry" after rinsing, therefore leaving as much of the antiparasitic properties as possible. Hopefully, this will repel parasites from moving onto the pet or kill them if they do. Always try to choose an antiparasitic shampoo that has a quality cleansing base. It is recommended that the face and head area be shampooed first. Care should be taken not to get these products in the eyes or mouth.

POWDERS Powders contain many of the same active ingredients as shampoos. The dog is liberally dusted with the product and then the powder is worked into the coat by brushing or rubbing against the grain of the coat. Powders kill fleas, lice, and *Cheyletiella* mites rapidly if applied in adequate concentrations. Ticks may be killed, but in most cases they seem resistant to the effects of powder. As long as the powder remains in the coat, its activity continues to protect the dog. However, with normal movement, most of the powder falls from the coat in a few days and reapplication is necessary. Powders are generally used when a problem is present, rather than as a preventative. They are especially popular in cats and puppies.

SPRAYS Insecticidal sprays are both very useful and very popular today. They contain a wide range of ingredients with various durations of activity. Additionally, they can be used to eliminate a current problem or applied as a preventative. While many are labeled for use against fleas, ticks, lice, and mites, they are usually used against fleas. There are some that are labeled specifically to use against ticks and, because of their formulations, are much more useful than the typical flea and tick varieties where ticks are a problem.

Sprays should be applied around the head and neck first and then over the rest of the body. Care should be taken not to get any of these products in the eyes or mouth. In long-haired breeds, it improves the efficacy of sprays to brush the dog against the grain of the hair coat during or immediately after application. This distributes the spray and its ingredients into the deeper layers of the coat.

Sprays can be water, alcohol, or oil based. Water bases are usually preferred as they have few, if any, harmful effects on the coat or skin. Many veterinarians and groomers dislike the alcohol based products, as it is believed that they tend to dry the skin and coat. Oil based products retain the insecticidal ingredients for a longer period of time on the animal, but are sticky and tend to attract dirt.

POUR-ONS These products are applied to a small area on the surface of the animal's skin. Following application, the active ingredients are absorbed through the skin in a brief period of time. They are then distributed by the blood system throughout the body. They are used to both repel and kill fleas, ticks, lice, and *Cheyletiella* mites that feed on the dog. They basically work the same as dips but are much easier to apply. Additionally, they generally do not have the offensive odor associated with dips, nor do they dry out the skin as is often noted with dips. Pour-ons have become very, very popular in the last few years because of the introduction of a single product, Defend-Exspot by Cooper Laboratories. To apply pour-ons, the hair is spread apart to expose the skin and the product is applied directly to the skin. This is usually done on a small area on top of the shoulders.

DIPS These solutions are used effectively against numerous ectoparasites. They are mostly formulated in strengths that not only kill the parasites present on the animal, but have residual activity lasting for a week or two. Their ingredients are generally absorbed through the skin. Some parasites, especially certain mites, are more susceptible to dips than other topical preparations.

Although the term "dip" implies that the entire animal is immersed in the solution, this is rarely the case. Typically, the dog is placed in a tub and first soaked in warm water with a sponge or sprayer. Next, while wearing rubber gloves, the individual uses a sponge to repeatedly soak the skin and hair coat of the animal with the dip solution. As the solution drips off the animal into the tub, it is soaked back up with the sponge and applied again until the coat is thoroughly saturated. As with a shampoo, it is best to start with the head and use caution to avoid getting solution in the eyes or mouth. Following the dipping, it is important that the animal "drip dry" so that the active ingredients soak in and dry on the animal's skin.

CHEMICALLY TREATED COLLARS/MEDALLIONS Chemically treated collars and medallions that attach to the dog's existing collar have continued to gain in popularity. They are made with several different active ingredients and different purposes. They are all impregnated with a chemical that is slowly emitted from the collar or medallion. The most common are the "flea and tick" combination varieties. These are best used as preventatives rather than when an infestation is already present. As would be expected, they are much more effective against fleas than the more resistant ticks.

There are collars made especially for use against ticks that contain specific agents to which ticks are more susceptible. Fleas are affected very little by collars that are labeled specifically for ticks. Additionally, there are collars that are made specifically against fleas that prevent their eggs from hatching. These may or may not affect adult fleas but rather limit the future populations.

Reactions to collars are actually quite rare. Most veterinarians feel that it is good practice to open the new collar and let it hang for a day or two to allow any excess insecticide present on the surface of the collar a chance to evaporate before being placed on the dog. *In many cases, a redness on the animal's skin that develops directly under the collar is actually an allergic reaction to the plastic and not the insecticidal preparations.* Many of these same dogs will develop a similar lesion on their mouths if fed with plastic food and water dishes. Collars should be fitted to the individual dog with any excess cut off and discarded.

ELECTRONIC COLLARS/MEDALLIONS   These tiny battery powered collars are used to repel fleas and ticks from dogs and cats. They produce a high frequency sound, inaudible to the human ear but supposedly very irritating to adult fleas, causing them to jump off or stay away from the dog without feeding. The efficacy of these products is difficult to ascertain but many owners believe they are very effective. They cause no known harmful effects to the dog. Many owners prefer them because they contain no potentially harmful chemicals.

ORAL PREPARATIONS   There are several products cleared and labeled for use in dogs. These are taken orally with the active ingredients being absorbed by the intestinal tract and spread throughout the body by the bloodstream. Fleas, depending on the ingredient, are either killed when they feed or are "chemically sterilized" and affected so their eggs cannot hatch.

Other oral preparations are also used that are not cleared for use on arthropod parasites. An example of this would be the ivermectin products that are commonly found in canine heartworm preventative medications and large animal (i.e., farm animals such as cattle and horses) wormers. Although not cleared for these uses, they are often administered orally in the treatment of various mite and lice species.

TREATMENT METHODS FOR THE HOME, YARD, AND KENNEL

Since certain ectoparasites spend a portion of their lives off of the dog, *it is important that the environment surrounding the pet also be treated to control these species.* Measures are directed at free living adults and/or immature life stages of the parasite. With some ectoparasitic organisms, this may involve over 85 percent of the total number that potentially affect the pet!

HOUSEHOLD SPRAYS   These are typically used after an infestation of fleas or ticks has occurred. They are rarely used in a preventative fashion. The sprays come in a wide range of ingredients that are often formulated to give them a prolonged residual activity. They may be designed to kill the parasites on contact and/or arrest the development of eggs or larvae.

Household sprays are applied on and under furniture, near baseboards and corners, and in other areas where the aerosol produced by foggers may not reach adequate concentrations.

CARPET POWDERS   These products are dusted into the carpet to kill parasitic forms that may remain hidden there for a long time. These are very similar to or identical to powders that are placed directly on the pet. The powders may be left in the carpet or, in some cases, applied and then vacuumed up after a specified time. In cases in which a severe infestation of the home has occurred, these products can be very useful.

FOGGERS   Timed-release aerosol foggers have become very popular today, especially after the home has become infested with fleas. They do have some effect on other arthropods but they are rarely used with these organisms in mind. Their formulation is designed to kill adult and most immature stages of the parasite. Some also contain ingredients that prevent the more resistant stages, such as eggs, from developing further. Like many anti-ectoparasitic products, foggers often contain claims on the label that a one-time use eliminates all problems for the season. This is rarely the case. In the authors' experience, a second fogging of the home two to four weeks after the initial treatment is sometimes necessary to really eliminate a problem.

YARD SPRAYS   These are similar to the sprays used on the pet or within the home but are usually of a stronger formulation or one more suited to outdoor use. They typically come premixed in a bottle that attaches to a garden hose, and are applied to the grass or kennel. Remove pets before use and allow the preparation to dry before animals are returned to the area.

BIOLOGICAL TREATMENTS   In the last few years a new non-chemical treatment to eradicate fleas has been developed for use both within the home and outdoors. These sprays and powders contain microscopically small worms called nematodes that attack developing flea larvae. Although they have been approved for use, few people have experience with them because of their newness. Initial reports on these products are very good. Many people prefer them because they replace potentially harmful chemicals.

ACTIVE INGREDIENTS OF PRODUCTS USED AGAINST ECTOPARASITES

As we shall see, there are numerous different products used against ectoparasites. To make it easier to understand, better explain the problems encountered with the different active ingredients, and note the complications that may arise because of interactions between different products, we will group them together by their chemical properties and/or actions. The vast majority of these compounds will have some effect on the pet. These are not detectable by observation in most cases and only rarely are serious side effects encountered. Still, owners should understand the potential problems and how to recognize them.

Pyrethrins and Pyrethroids
Pyrethrins are natural insecticides found in the flowers of the chrysanthemum plant. *Many flea and tick products that are labeled as "all natural" contain pyrethrins.*

Pyrethrins are very popular because they have the ability, at adequate concentrations, to rapidly kill fleas, lice, and *Cheyletiella* mites. Ticks are more resistant to their usage. These factors, plus the fact that they are very safe in dogs and cats, account for their popularity of use today. Pyrethrins at lower concentrations (0.05 percent concentration) are one of the few products sometimes labeled for use on pregnant dogs or very young puppies. Additionally, all of the pyrethrins possess the ability to repel these same ectoparasites, further protecting the dog.

The disadvantage of the natural pyrethrins is that they have little residual activity. They are quickly broken down by such things as sunlight. After a few days following application, little insecticidal activity remains. **Piperonyl butoxide,** a synergist, is often added to pyrethrin products to increase their effectiveness, duration of activity, and strength. Other processes such as microencapsulation also extend the effective life of pyrethrins.

Today, **synthetic pyrethrins** have been developed and can be easily manufactured. These are referred to as **pyrethroids.** They have a much longer duration of activity, often labeled for up to fourteen days or longer, as they are more resistant to the environmental factors which break down the chemical structure of the naturally occurring pyrethrins. They are more effective against ticks than are the pyrethrins. Although they have a low incidence of toxicity in dogs, they are usually not as safe as natural pyrethrins. *Permethrin* is the one most commonly used in preparations designed for use in dogs. Others are *fenvalerate, resmethrin, allethrin,* and *tetramethrin.*

Pyrethrins and pyrethroids are found in shampoos, powders, foggers, dips, and sprays used both on the pet and in the environment. Many preparations of pyrethrins will have a synergist, piperonyl butoxide, incorporated into the formulation. Synergists aid the effectiveness of the product by increasing its strength and the length of time that it remains active.

Pyrethrins and pyrethroids are very safe and side effects are rarely observed in the dog. Some animals may be more sensitive to these products than others and problems are generally associated with nervous system stimulation. After topical application, these compounds may pass through the skin, be inhaled, or be ingested when the dog licks itself. Problems most commonly noted are excess salivation or drooling, vomiting, diarrhea, refusing to eat, muscle twitching, and in rare cases staggering, seizures, and subnormal body temperature. If the products are used as labeled, however, any of these signs would be very, very rare. *Problems are most likely to occur when several different pyrethrins or pyrethroids are simultaneously used* on a dog. As would be expected, toxic problems are also likely to occur when compounds from several different groups of insecticides are used simultaneously.

Rotenone

Isolated from plants, **rotenone** (Goodwinol Ointment, Ear Mitecide by Vedco) is another anti-ectoparasitic that is often listed as being "all natural." Specifically, it comes from the root of the derris plant. It can be found in products labeled for use against fleas, ticks, ear mites, and different forms of mange.

Although considered to be very safe if used according to label instructions, unwanted or toxic reactions are more common with rotenone than with pyrethrin/pyrethroid usage. The signs are similar; i.e., nervous system stimulation leading to drooling, vomiting, diarrhea, and muscle twitching.

D-Limonene

This substance is isolated from the peel of citrus fruits. It is found in different formulations such as shampoos, dips, and sprays, and these are usually labeled for fleas and ticks. In the authors' experience, d-limonene is typically not as effective as the pyrethrin/pyrethroids or rotenone. It is labeled for use both to kill fleas and ticks and also to repel them. In dogs, d-limonene is very safe if used as directed. If used at excessive levels, toxicity can develop. Clinical signs reported would be excessive drooling, vomiting, diarrhea, muscle twitching, staggering, and in extremely rare cases, an abnormally low body temperature.

CHOLINESTERASE INHIBITORS

The **carbamates** and **organophosphates** are classified as cholinesterase inhibitors and are found in a wide range of anti-ectoparasitic treatments. These chemicals interfere with the functioning of the parasite's nervous system. They have the ability to quickly kill the various parasites on contact and are also used to prevent new infestations. They are found in collars, sprays, etc., and are very effective at these tasks. While they do not have the wide safety range that is found with the pyrethrins and pyrethroids, they are very popular in canine medicine today.

Carbamates are routinely used to prevent or treat ectoparasitic infestations in the dog. Some of the more common ones are **carbaryl, propoxur, bendiocarb, carbofuran,** and **aldicarb.** These are found in numerous formulations under various brand names. **Organophosphates** are used in various medications as well as many anti-ectoparasitic preparations. Examples are **chlorpyrifos** (Dursban, found in flea collars, sprays, foggers, lawn sprays, etc.), **chlorfenvinphos, dichlorvos** (Vapona and also in the wormer Task), **fenthion** (Pro-Spot), **phosmet** (Paramite Dip), **malathion,** and **cythioate** (Proban, which is a tablet taken orally to protect against fleas).

Adverse reactions are not uncommon with the cholinesterase inhibitors. Most of the products are absorbed internally into the dog. However, if used as directed, problems rarely occur. Use of this class of drugs should be avoided or at least watched closely in the sighthounds (such as the Greyhound) because of their sensitivities. The same would be true for sick or debilitated animals. However, if one uses more than the label or common sense would dictate, unwanted side effects can occur in any dog. The same can happen if someone picks several different cholinesterase inhibitors and uses them simultaneously. For example, if the dog is dipped, the coat is sprayed heavily, Proban tablets are administered, a new flea collar is put on, and a premise spray inside the home and a lawn spray are used all on the same day or over a very short period of time, there is a very real potential for adverse reactions. This is when problems with cholinesterase inhibitors occur in the dog—too many different products from the same class used excessively at the same time. The animal's nervous system is overwhelmed by these products and the nerves repeatedly fire in an uncontrolled fashion.

Clinical signs of toxicity with these preparations are somewhat similar to those seen with the previously discussed anti-ectoparasitic products. Most affected animals will drool excessively; vomit; stagger; and have diarrhea, constricted pupils, muscle twitching, seizures, and even an elevated body temperature.

INSECT GROWTH INHIBITORS

In the last decade, usage of this group of medications has grown dramatically. They have little, if any, effect on the adult insect. Their chemical makeup is formulated so that they either kill or prevent the development of the offspring of the treated adult insects. Since they do not eliminate the adult forms of the ectoparasites, they should and can safely be used with any of the previously mentioned products to eliminate a current problem.

Examples of these insect growth inhibitors are **nylar** (Drs. Foster and Smith Multi-Stage Fogger), **methoprene** (Precor, found in Ovitrol Plus), **fenoxycarb** (X-O-TROL foggers), and **lufeneron** (Program tablets). Nylar, methoprene and fenoxycarb are formulated in many different sprays, collars, foggers, etc., for use on the animal and in the environment. They have hormonal activity that acts on the larval stages of the parasites, preventing them from developing into adults. The growth inhibitors have no effect on the adult fleas, but these products can be used simultaneously with those that do. Some products that contain growth inhibitors also contain other previously discussed ingredients whose action is directed at the adult ectoparasites. This provides a two-step defense against the parasites. An example would be Ovitrol Plus flea spray, which contains both methoprene and pyrethrin.

Program tablets, which contain lufeneron, are given on a monthly basis. They prevent the flea eggs produced by adults feeding on a treated dog from hatching into larvae. This prevents the production of future generations. The product does nothing to repel or eliminate the adult fleas and should therefore be thought of only as part of an overall program to prevent or eliminate flea problems in dogs.

For the dog, the growth inhibitors are very, very safe. Few side effects or adverse reactions have been recorded. Their hormonal activity does not affect dogs.

Amitraz

Amitraz is utilized against mites and ticks in canine medicine. It is found in anti-tick collars (Preventic) and dips used primarily against demodectic mange (Mitaban). It functions by inhibiting the enzyme **monoamine oxidase** in the parasite's metabolism. Since this mechanism of action is totally different from the other anti-ectoparasites discussed in this chapter, it can be used in conjunction with them, providing an additive effect.

In the authors' experience, few unwanted side effects have been noted with the use of these products. The most commonly noted clinical signs of toxicosis are lethargy and lack of coordination. Others are a slower heart rate, vomiting, diarrhea, and elevations or suppressions of body temperature. These are most commonly seen if the dog is allowed to chew on or eat a collar treated with amitraz. These collars should be fitted to the dog, with any excess cut off and discarded.

Ivermectin

This product has become very popular in the last decade in the treatment of *many* parasitic disorders. Originally developed as a livestock wormer, today it is found in products labeled for use in canines. Most of these are monthly heartworm preventatives (e.g., Heartgard). Additionally, ivermectin is used to treat many ectoparasitic diseases. Although no products are yet labeled for these uses, many veterinarians routinely use the cattle wormer Ivomec to successfully treat various forms of mite and louse infestations. Ear and nasal mites, as well as the more generalized forms such as sarcoptic mange and *Cheyletiella,* are usually easily eliminated with these treatments. Many practitioners also use ivermectin as part of the treatment of demodectic mange.

While ivermectin has been used in these off-label fashions for several years, few problems have been encountered. Generally, this medication is not used in Collies or Collie crosses when used at these dosages, which are higher than those required for heartworm protection. They have a much higher sensitivity to the product, which crosses into their central nervous system. Whenever this occurs, it may cause ataxia, seizures, coma, and even death, regardless of breed. Significantly, *there is no antidote to ivermectin toxicosis at this time.* Additionally, *ivermectin does not interact with other medications.*

Cancer Therapeutics

Cancer is best described as an abnormal growth of cells. These abnormal cells may simply cause an erosion or loss of normal cells, as in some skin cancers, or they may grow in clumps or clusters forming tumors often referred to as growths, masses, or nodules.

A cancer is usually, but not always, named for the organ(s) it invades or where the cancer originated. Such terms may include: **bone cancer, skin cancer, lung cancer, liver cancer, intestinal cancer, brain cancer, uterine cancer, mammary cancer,** etc. Scientifically, clinicians usually refer to cancers by cell type rather than organ involvement. Examples would include terms such as **adenocarcinoma, squamous cell carcinoma, malignant melanoma, lymphosarcoma,** etc. Some forms of cancer are more severe than others.

A *malignant* cancer is one that is life-threatening, as the abnormal cells cause extreme local destruction and are often likely to spread **(metastasize)** to other organs or areas of the body. *Benign* cancers are not life-threatening and generally do not spread or cause extensive local crowding of abnormal cells. The suffix "oma" may denote a benign tumor while the ending "sarcoma" or "carcinoma" usually suggests a more malignant form. An example would be a tumor of glandular tissue, called an adenoma if benign and an adenocarcinoma if malignant. The nomenclature is not exact and many more names and terms can apply to various cancers.

From an owner's standpoint, the nomenclature is not as important as: How serious is it? Can it be treated? How? And of course, what can be expected?

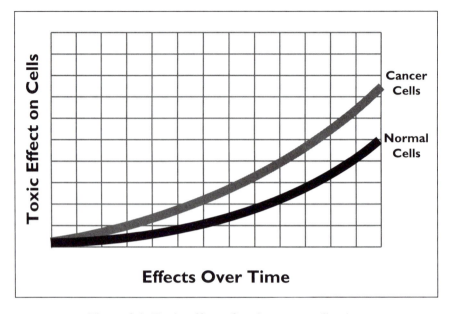

**Figure 9-1: Toxic effect of anticancer medication
on normal cells and cancer cells.**

Some cancers, especially benign forms, may require no treatment. Others may require surgical removal, cryosurgery (freezing), radiation therapy, drug therapy (chemotherapy), or a combination of the above. This chapter, however, is about chemotherapy and the various commonly used drugs that may be prescribed.

The selection of the proper drugs for use in a chemotherapeutic program is based on such things as: cancer type, malignant or benign, and the age and condition of the patient. The goal of therapy is to kill or inhibit the growth of the cancerous cells while causing little harm to the normal cells of the body. *Almost all cells of the body are in some way affected by anticancer drugs, usually in some harmful manner.* Cancer cells are more affected, however, because of their rapid growth and division, selective uptake of the drug, or their sensitivities to its action. The drugs usually do not cure the disease but may only slow its spread or place it into remission for a period of time. In most malignant canine forms the cancer still leads to the death of the animal.

Below is a list of the drugs more commonly used to treat cancer in the canine.

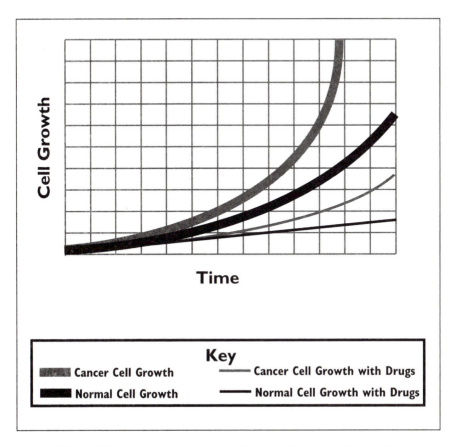

Figure 9-2: Anticancer drugs and their effect on cell growth.

Cyclophosphamide
Cyclophosphamide (Cytoxan) is occasionally dispensed in tablet form to be administered for a period of several months to treat various forms of cancers including, but not limited to, cancers of the lymph nodes, bladder, mammary glands, and lungs. Side effects may include hemorrhage, nausea, vomiting, hair loss, and suppression of the number of red and white blood cells.

Vincristine
Vincristine (Oncovin) has been widely used in the treatment of cancer, especially those of the lymph nodes. It is commonly utilized in combination with other anticancer drugs. Side effects may include

suppression of white blood cell production, hair loss, mouth ulcers, seizures, and liver upsets.

Glucocorticoids (Prednisone, Prednisolone)

Prednisone has been shown to inhibit the growth and reproduction of certain types of cancer cells arising from the lymph glands. The glucocorticoids such as prednisone are commonly used in combination with other cancer-treating drugs such as vincristine. Side effects may include increased thirst and urination, loss of hair, water retention, gastric ulcers, and cataracts. These side effects are not seen with lower doses. However, the higher doses used to treat cancers may produce these unwanted results. In some cancers in the dog such as those of the lymph nodes, prednisone may be the only product used. It will shrink these tumors and slow the progression of the disease.

Doxorubicin

Doxorubicin (Adriamycin) is occasionally utilized to treat cancers of the thyroid, lymph, and mammary glands. Toxicities include loss of appetite, vomiting, diarrhea, nausea, and anemia.

CHAPTER 10
Steroids

Steroids comprise one of the most beneficial groups of medications in veterinary medicine today.

It is easy to say that steroids are often misunderstood and sometimes controversial. A complete description would have to include the facts that they actually cure nothing, have no set or consistent dosage, are potentially harmful in many situations, but are in fact produced naturally by the body. Many owners go to their veterinarians on a routine basis for steroidal therapy for their pets, while others become angry if these drugs are even mentioned as part of a treatment.

Today, many cats and dogs are either alive or are able to live longer and more comfortably because of the beneficial effects of steroids. These medications have one of the widest ranges of use of any class of drugs. They are found in every veterinary clinic, in every conceivable type of preparation, for use in every possible way. Below are two typical case histories.

It's August and a dog has started chewing on its feet and scratching its sides. It happens every year, usually starting within a few days of the same calendar date. It finally reaches the point where the dog either mutilates itself or scratches through the night and keeps the owner awake. The veterinarian administers an injection and dispenses some pills for the owner to give over a three-week period. The doctor tells the client the problem is an allergy to pollen and that the medications are a form of cortisone or steroids. The signs are gone within two days. The dog finishes up the pills and the condition doesn't return until the following August.

In a second case, a severely debilitated dog with a long term viral illness fails to respond to therapy. The disease continues to take its toll. The owner and veterinarian have reached the point where, unless the condition can be turned around, they will choose to humanely put the animal to sleep. In this case, due to lack of exercise and caloric intake, the animal has wasted away, with muscles atrophied or shrunken in size. Their ability to function is greatly impaired. The dog has little or no appetite and will only eat if it is personally hand fed by the owner. Even though the case has reached the point where the virus is no longer present in the animal's body, the dog is going to die (either on its own or at the hands of the veterinarian) simply because it has lost the physical ability and mental attitude to recover. At this point, the animal is given a steroid, an uncommon one; the condition reverses itself over a three-week period. Mentally and physically the dog's health is much improved, and the medication is discontinued and the animal goes on to return to normal vigor.

Most dog owners consider steroids to be drugs manufactured by pharmaceutical firms or possibly isolated from plants or other sources in the environment. However, all mammals constantly produce their own supply of these substances within their bodies. One of the first steroids discovered was **cortisol,** which is naturally produced by the adrenal glands of all animals. The adrenal glands are small, paired structures, one lying in front of each kidney. They produce three different types of steroids: **mineralocorticoids, sex steroids,** and the **glucocorticoids.**

Mineralocorticoids get their name from the fact that they have the responsibility of maintaining the levels of the minerals sodium and potassium in the body, and because they are produced by the cortex of the adrenal glands. Through their effect on sodium and potassium, as well as other actions, they conserve or maintain the body's concentration of water at a near constant level. Mineralocorticoids exert most of their effect on the kidneys, causing parts of these organs to selectively excrete excess potassium in the urine and at the same time conserve or retain sodium. These actions maintain the concentrations of these electrolytes within a very narrow range that is compatible with life. The use of the mineralocorticoids or their synthetically produced imitations in veterinary medicine is much less common than the other two forms of steroids. Therefore they will not be covered in this text.

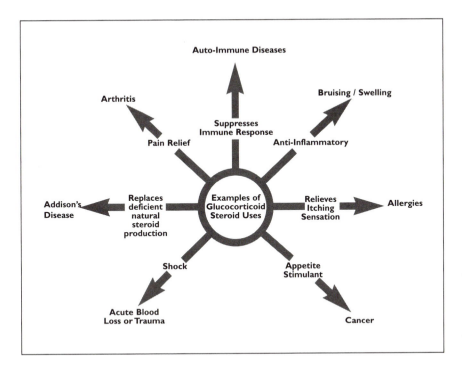

Figure 10-1: Reasons for glucocorticoid steroid use and specific medical conditions.

The second steroid type produced by these glands is the **sex steroids.** Examples of these are the female hormones estrogen and progesterone and the male androgens such as testosterone. These same substances are also produced in much greater quantities by the ovaries in the female and the testicles in the male. The androgens are the group that are sometimes referred to as anabolic steroids. Although they have accepted uses in medicine today, they often get considerable publicity when they are abused by athletes to increase their strength and abilities unethically.

They are totally different in activity and usage from the glucocorticoids or mineralocorticoids. The anabolic uses of the sex steroids will be discussed later in this chapter, while their use in reproduction will be covered with the other male and female hormonal products in chapter 21, on reproductive systems drugs.

The previously mentioned **cortisol** belongs to the **glucocorticoid** group. The members of this group get their name because they affect glucose metabolism and are produced by the cortex section of the adrenal glands. *The glucocorticoids are the predominant steroids used in veterinary medicine.* These naturally occurring steroids cause proteins (e.g., muscles) and lipids (e.g., body fats) to be chemically broken down and converted into glucose. This is why the glucocorticoids are also referred to as the "catabolic" steroids. Catabolism means to break down large molecules into smaller ones. Additionally, the glucocorticoids also cause carbohydrates stored in the form of glycogen to be converted back to glucose and deposited into the circulating blood. There it is available to all the body's tissues. To break down the proteins or fats of the body may seem harmful to the animal, but remember that glucose is the main energy source for all of the body's activities. The vast majority of the glucose that the body utilizes comes directly from the diet or stored glycogen, but in emergency situations it can be derived from its own protein and lipids. It is generally thought that the glucocorticoids only cause this to occur to a significant degree during periods of exceptional need.

Glucocorticoids also suppress inflammatory processes within the body. A bruise, bee sting, sprained ankle, bacterial infection, or arthritis are just a few examples of inflammation within a dog's body. Inflammation is specifically defined as an area of the body characterized by redness, swelling, heat, and pain, often with impaired function. The warmth and redness seen in these affected tissues comes from an increase in the number and size of blood vessels within the area. The swelling **(edema)** is caused by free fluid within the tissues and also the engorged blood vessels. All of these changes are brought on by physical trauma and/or irritants within the tissues. The pain is caused by the swelling, by harmful substances putting pressure on, or by stimulating the local nerve fibers. The loss of function can be caused by pain or the simple inability of the body to move or act correctly.

THE ANDROGEN GROUP—ANABOLIC STEROIDS

These compounds are related to the male hormone **testosterone.** They are referred to as the **anabolic steroids** because they cause the formation of new proteins. As we stated before, they are often abused by athletes trying to increase strength and muscle mass.

Their use in canine medicine, while infrequent, is related to these and similar properties.

Anabolic steroids come in liquid forms for injection and tablets for oral administration. Two of the most commonly used in canine medicine are **stanozolol** (Winstrol-V) and **nandrolone** (DecaDurabolin).

Animals that have been sick for a long time or who have been through severe, debilitating injuries often have generalized weakness and atrophied muscles. In some, this has progressed to the point where the animals can no longer walk or even stand. Their bodies are just too run down and, without some outside stimulation, they simply may give up the will to live.

Anabolic steroids are sometimes useful in these situations. The therapy may take several weeks. The medications can be most helpful if the veterinarian recognizes the condition before too much strength is lost. Anabolic steroids assist the body in regaining its muscle mass by building new proteins, which are the primary constituent of muscle fibers. Additionally, they help strengthen existing muscles.

In some of these same cases, anabolic steroids are frequently used to stimulate the debilitated or recovering patient's appetite. To achieve this effect usually requires several days to several weeks of therapy for significant changes.

The anabolic steroids are also useful in treating certain types of anemia. Anemia is the term used to describe lower than normal numbers of **red blood cells (RBCs).** In certain cases where the bone marrow has stopped producing new RBCs, administration of anabolic steroids will stimulate this system and bring the number of these cells back to normal levels. They also are known to stimulate the production of **white blood cells** (the blood cells associated with the immune response) and **platelets** (tiny cells in blood that assist in clotting) to a lesser degree. In these situations, the anabolic steroids are useful only in increasing the numbers of these cells. *They do not increase the ability of the cells to function.*

Kidney failure often brings on anemia because these organs may fail to produce the substance **erythropoietin.** Its normal function is to monitor the level of RBCs in the body and to stimulate the bone marrow to increase production when RBC numbers are too low. In its absence, anabolic steroids are often useful in reversing the effects of this anemia. They do not cause new erythropoietin to be produced; they only replace its function.

In many situations, the anabolic steroids fail to provide the benefits described here. Regardless of which particular product is used, it is often impossible to reverse the condition present. These are not miracle drugs that can save every debilitated or severely ill patient, but in some they can help.

As stated, these medications are closely related to testosterone and many of the problems associated with their usage are brought on by the normal actions of the male hormones. They can cause cessation of heat cycles and imitation of mounting behavior in females. In males, they have been found to increase the incidence of prostate disease and certain hernias and tumors that are caused by normal testosterone levels in older male dogs. Normal sperm production is often disrupted, with few new cells being formed. None of these problems are considered significant in these cases, as many of the patients are already in a life or death situation.

Anabolic steroids also cause water retention and this can cause additional complications in kidney or heart failure patients. These products also increase the absorption of calcium by the intestinal tract and cause the kidneys to retain calcium during normal urine production. Both of these actions lead to excessively high calcium levels in the blood which can be disastrous to normal heart function. This can be quickly fatal in those with already failing hearts.

GLUCOCORTICOIDS—THE CATABOLIC STEROIDS

When steroids are mentioned in the treatment of animal disorders, they are almost always of the **glucocorticoid** type. Naturally occurring **cortisol** is not used, but is replaced by others that can be produced more economically. Their use is generally intended to directly or indirectly reduce inflammation and irritation or to decrease the body's natural response against itself or outside stimuli. Examples of these products would be **hydrocortisone, prednisone, prednisolone, dexamethasone** (Azium), **betamethasone** (Betasone), **triamcinolone** (Vetalog), **methylated prednisolone** (Cortisate-20, Depo-Medrol, and Medrol), and others. Generic formulations are very common and are available in topical or systemic forms.

Exactly how glucocorticoids (either those produced naturally or given as a medication) reduce inflammation is not exactly understood at this time. It is believed that they stabilize individual cells and their internal structures so that they do not release the substances which initiate or perpetuate the irritation, pain, and swelling referred to as **inflammation.** Glucocorticoids probably also inhibit those substances already within the affected area. The ability of glucocorticoid steroids to control or suppress inflammation is the most common reason for their use in medicine.

Glucocorticoids also decrease the body's response to substances, cells, or organisms that are, or are perceived as, potentially harmful or foreign. In a healthy dog, the immune system correctly recognizes disease-causing bacterial, viral, or fungal organisms as foreign invaders. It attacks them with white blood cells and large protein molecules called antibodies. This is totally beneficial to the individual. However, in an animal affected by an autoimmune disease such as **lupus,** the immune system mistakenly sees parts of its own body as foreign and tries to destroy them. In the example of lupus, the system specifically attacks its own blood cells, kidneys, and joint surfaces. In the absence of medical treatment, this usually leads to the animal's death. In either of these cases, *the glucocorticoids eliminate the immune system's ability to see particles as abnormal, or decreases the response against them.* This suppression of the immune system can be either beneficial or an unwanted side effect of glucocorticoids, depending on the situation in which they are used.

Before we discuss specific uses of these products, we need to stress several important points.

- Glucocorticoids, with the exception of one condition, are unable to cure or eliminate any of the diseases they are used to treat.
- The beneficial actions of these steroids only suppress the harmful effects of the disorders while they are being used. As soon as these medications are withdrawn, the problem may reappear.

They can, in some cases, suppress the body's actions long enough for tissues to heal correctly on their own, but the steroids play no part in the actual repair. In other cases, they may be used against seasonal allergies and the animal is taken off the drugs only after the irritating agent (the allergen) is gone for that year. In the example given above, they did not cure the problem but rather only reduced the body's reactions (e.g., allergy to weed pollen). Sometimes the disease is cured by other means and the steroids can be discontinued. The only example of steroids actually reversing or bringing a disorder under control by themselves is the example of hypovolemic shock, which will be discussed later.

- The problems or side effects associated with glucocorticoid usage can occur immediately or long after the drugs have been discontinued. It is important that both owners and veterinarians be aware of them so they are quickly recognized. In most cases, much can be done to prevent or correct them.

  Increased water consumption and increased urination are two of the most common side effects of glucocorticoid usage. Although it can be quite disconcerting to the owner of a dog that lives predominately in the home, it is not by itself a serious problem. Glucocorticoids increase the activity of the **glomeruli,** which are the filtration units of the kidneys. This causes the animal to excrete higher levels of urine. The loss stimulates thirst in an attempt to replace lost fluids. These actions may increase water consumption and urination to the point that the animal can control neither one. Such signs can be observed within hours of initiating steroid therapy if the initial dosages were too high for the individual animal to tolerate. When long-acting injectable forms are used at excessive levels, increased water consumption and urination can continue for several weeks!

- During use, and for a period thereafter, these steroids will suppress the immune system to some degree and therefore make the animal more susceptible to viral, bacterial, or fungal diseases. To overcome this problem, antibiotics or other medications are frequently given concurrently with steroid therapy to protect the animal from opportunistic organisms taking advantage of the suppressed immune system.

- They will alter the animal's metabolism of protein and can easily lead to muscular weakness or atrophy. With consistent and long term use, the signs of this can become quite apparent. The abdominal muscles may weaken, causing the animal to have a sagging or pendulous abdomen. Additional strength can be lost from the legs, causing the animal to have difficulty raising itself after lying down, climbing steps, or walking long distances.

- Steroids will also alter glucose metabolism, and their use in a diabetic animal can be disastrous. As excessive glucose is produced, the blood sugar elevates abnormally and the animal's need for insulin increases dramatically. During pregnancy, steroid use can easily cause an abortion. Some animals will also seem more lethargic or tired while on these medications; others may show increased appetites.
- The glucocorticoids also affect calcium utilization in the body. Not only do they cause less calcium to be absorbed through the intestinal wall, but they also cause the kidneys to excrete excessive calcium through the urine. Combined, they cause the body to steal from its own major storage site of calcium, the skeleton. As it selectively removes calcium from the bones for use in other areas, the bones become weaker and could be more prone to fracture. Although the biochemical pathways in which this can occur are easy to understand, bone problems associated with steroid usage in dogs are very, very rare.

We must stress that by monitoring the dosage and response of the patient, all of the above side effects of glucocorticoid usage are usually easily prevented and the desired beneficial results obtained. Most of these problems, with the exception of induced abortion, are easy to recognize and quickly reversed when steroid usage is decreased or discontinued.

However, possibly the most serious and life-threatening side effect of steroid therapy is not always so easy to recognize initially. After use is discontinued, or during prolonged use, steroids can have severe effects on the adrenal glands. The brain and the pituitary gland routinely monitor the levels of the mineralocorticoids and glucocorticoids within the body. When their concentrations are low, they signal the adrenal glands to produce more, or vice versa.

This system can be fooled by long term administration of glucocorticoids, confusing the synthetic products with those naturally produced by its own adrenal glands. In the presence of higher than normal levels of these compounds, it senses no need for further production and may turn off the adrenal glands completely.

Unfortunately, when the medications are later discontinued, the glands may fail to re-initiate normal levels of production. This leaves the body totally without or with greatly reduced concentrations of its own natural regulating steroids. This condition is referred to as **Addison's disease** and it usually requires expensive lifelong therapy to save the animal's life. In other cases, after therapy is discontinued the adrenal glands may not respond correctly to feedback regulation, go out of control, and release large quantities of cortisol. This leads to the equally serious **Cushing's disease,** which also requires expensive lifelong therapy to control.

The above list of potential side effects may frighten the average dog owner. They are, however, the exception. *The vast majority of all cases in which steroids are used provide great benefit to the dog without any side effects occurring!* When serious problems do occur, it is usually in cases in which steroids were administered over very long periods of time or at excessive doses. Large single doses or short term use at normal levels rarely, if ever, causes a serious problem unless there is some pre-existing condition such as diabetes, pregnancy, or heart disease.

DOSAGE

From the veterinarian's point of view, an additional problem with steroid therapy is that none of the products or the disease syndromes treated have exact dosages. It varies with each condition and each patient. Although dosages are listed in appendix I, these are only rough guidelines. As with an anesthetic agent, the goal is to use only the minimum amount necessary to produce the desired effect. Two animals weighing exactly the same and having the same disorder may require very different dosages of steroids to control the condition and/or prevent side effects. Veterinarians are constantly doing a balancing act between these two extremes of steroid usage. When an animal is sent home under the observation of the owner, frequent communication with the veterinarian is necessary to describe how the disease is responding and how the patient is dealing with the medication. One of the first problems that owners will see at home will be excessive water consumption and urination. If side effects occur, then the dosage needs to be lowered, a different medication used, or possibly all steroid usage discontinued.

Additionally, the dosage for steroids usually changes with each patient over time. The animal is usually started at a high or "loading" dose for a few days, and is then dropped to a long term maintenance level. Finally, a reduced dosage is utilized that slowly

weans the animal's body off the medication. During the maintenance stage, it is preferred to use oral medications and give them
only every other day in the morning. This also reduces the chance
of suppressing the hypophyseal/pituitary gland feedback system on
the adrenal glands.

By gradually decreasing the level of steroids at the end of the
treatment, veterinarians greatly reduce or eliminate potential problems that can lead to Cushing's or Addison's by confusing the
regulatory feedback mechanisms described above. For a complete
listing of the dosages of the medications discussed in this chapter
and others, please refer to appendix I.

COMMON STEROIDS IN CANINE MEDICATION

As stated above, every veterinary clinic has numerous steroid medications, including injectable solutions; tablets; and topical preparations such as creams, ointments, or skin preparations. They may be
single formulas or mixed with other medications. Their most common use is to control or eliminate inflammation. Among other
things, they are also used to treat shock and, in the case of autoimmune diseases, they are prescribed to suppress immune systems
that are out of control.

Although other compounds could be listed, over 98 percent of
all steroids used in dogs are either **hydrocortisone, prednisone,
prednisolone, triamcinolone** (Vetalog), **methylprednisolone** (Depo-
Medrol and Medrol), **dexamethasone** (Azium), or **betamethasone**
(Betasone). We can easily classify the different medications by their
strength and time of effectiveness in the body. Many texts use the
naturally occurring cortisol as a standard. You can calculate the
amount of glucocorticoid activity as being directly proportional to
anti-inflammatory effects. That is to say, the higher the glucocorticoid activity, the greater its effect will be on suppressing inflammation and vice versa. Using this method, hydrocortisone has basically
the same glucocorticoid or anti-inflammatory strength as the natural cortisol. It is the weakest of the commonly used steroids. Prednisone and prednisolone are both three to four times stronger in
their anti-inflammatory effects as cortisol. They have been used for
decades and their action is often easier to predict than some of the
stronger preparations. Methylprednisolone and triamcinolone are

newer synthetics with about five to seven times the strength of cortisol in their glucocorticoid effects. Dexamethasone and betamethasone are the powerhouses of steroids. They are thirty to forty times more powerful than cortisol in their effect on inflammation.

As to the length of activity after a single injection, the relative glucocorticoid strength parallels the duration of action within the body. Cortisol and hydrocortisone only last for twelve hours or less. Prednisone, prednisolone, triamcinolone, and methylprednisolone last for twelve to thirty-six hours, while dexamethasone and betamethasone show activity for over forty-eight hours! This is only a true comparison when they are given by injection. If they are taken orally or formulated with other products that affect their breakdown and excretion from the body, the duration of action can be greatly increased. For example, Betasone is a combination betamethasone, specifically betamethasone diproprionate. When it is injected under the skin, the effects on the body are continuous and can easily last for up to three to six weeks. Depo-Medrol is a long-acting injectable form of methylprednisolone that lasts for two to five weeks.

Most veterinarians today prefer not to use the long-acting injectable products like Betasone or the similar methylprednisolone product Depo-Medrol. They are usually fine for a single injection but their repeated use in the same animal can cause suppression of the hypophyseal section of the brain and pituitary gland and other side effects. When long term therapy is being considered, it is much easier to use oral forms like the short-acting prednisone or prednisolone tablets on an every-other-day schedule. With tablets, the dosage can be quickly changed at any time. With long-acting injections, nothing can be done to alter the effect once the product is in the animal's body.

Animals that have suffered severe injuries, such as being hit by a car, attacked by another animal, or shot, usually slip into **hypovolemic shock.** They may not have lost large quantities of blood, but rather they go into a physiological state in which the large blood vessels within the abdomen and its organs dilate and the blood tends to stagnate or pool there. This is a defensive action by the body to prevent further loss and hopefully save its life. However, due to lack of fluid volume, the remainder of the animal's circulatory system goes into near total collapse. When they reach the veterinary hospital, these animals are immediately placed on intravenous fluids and large doses of steroids are administered intravenously. Within minutes or even seconds the signs of shock usually start to abate. These drugs cause the blood vessels within the abdomen to constrict, forcing the blood throughout the animal's body. The above signs are quickly reversed and if there are no other life-threatening problems, the animal quickly recovers. The steroids used are usually methylprednisolone products manufactured strictly for this purpose. They seem to work as fast or faster than any of the other steroids and are sold under such brand names as Cortisate-20, Solu-Delta-Cortef, etc.

Many hospitalized dogs are on steroids as part of a total therapeutic regime. As a component of their anti-inflammatory effect, steroids are excellent in reducing swelling and/or edema from the body's tissues. An example of this use would be in an animal that has ruptured a disc between the vertebrae in its back. The swollen, herniated disc puts pressure on the spinal cord and other nerve fibers in the area. This is painful and the pressure on the spinal cord prevents nerve impulses from passing between the brain and the rear part of the body. The animal may be unable to walk or control its colon or bladder. Severe damage to the spinal cord can lead to total paralysis or death. Although surgery is required in a small portion of these cases to relieve the pressure on the spinal cord, most of these dogs can be successfully handled with rest and steroids. The steroids, and this case it is often dexamethasone, are able to remove the swelling and fluid within the disc and surrounding tissues, thereby removing the pressure from the spinal cord. This allows the nerve fibers within it to function correctly. Given time, the disc shrinks back down and the steroids are slowly discontinued. Remember, the steroids do not "heal" the disc; they only reduce the swelling while it slowly returns to its normal size and shape.

Another typical example of steroid use removing inflammation can be seen with certain eye disorders. Often the **cornea** (the membrane or surface that a contact lens rests on) becomes cloudy following an injury or because of a disease called **pannus.** Instead of being perfectly clear, it is opaque from the cells and inflammatory material trapped within it. The animal's vision may be affected. Left untreated, this area would remain as is or even worsen. With this disorder, steroids are injected into the **sclera** or "white of the eye," or placed topically on the cornea. Slowly, the medication seeps out from the injection site into the surrounding tissues and removes the infiltration of cells, edema, and exudate from the cornea. Unfortunately, this doesn't cure the disease and the pannus lesions may return and require similar treatment again in the future.

A final but very different use of glucocorticoids in a hospital situation is for appetite stimulation. Animals that are recovering from or dealing with severe or long term illnesses often lose their appetite. These animals simply need a "pick-me-up" to get them started back on their food. This is not the same as when we use anabolic steroids; those are for long term usage. In the case described here, one injection of dexamethasone will usually be all that is necessary to stimulate the appetite. Once veterinarians get them to take that first meal, they usually continue to eat on their own.

When the dog is in the home, steroids have an even broader spectrum of uses. The principles are still the same, with their primary function reducing or controlling inflammation, but this includes a very wide range of medical conditions. They are also used to control the immune system, as with the autoimmune disorders.

The most common usage of steroids in the home is to control or decrease an animal's response to **allergies.** Some allergies will be seasonal, with the problem coming from exposure to pollen, flea bites, or molds. When dogs develop an allergy to something they *inhale* (e.g., pollen), or something that comes in *contact with* their skin (e.g., a flea bite or particular carpet fiber), or something they *eat* (e.g., beef by-products in their diet), the disease presents itself as a *skin disease.* Dogs with allergies scratch their sides, chew on their feet, and may have repeated ear infections because of increased wax production. The scratching and chewing is brought on by severe itching sensations. The allergy actually causes an inflammatory reaction within the skin in these areas. In the ears, the excessive wax production is caused by inflammation affecting the skin and the glands that are responsible for producing the wax. Rather than being at a single site, the inflammation is found over large areas of the body.

These types of allergies in the dog are treated in several ways. Some may be very seasonal in nature and the veterinarian may choose to give a single long-acting injection like Depo-Medrol or Betasone. The rationale for this is that the injection will last three to six weeks and by then the allergen will be gone from the environment. If it is expected to last longer than this, veterinarians would commonly give the dog an injection of a short-acting steroid like prednisone that would last for two to three days. This would be a "loading dose" to immediately "put the fire out." The client would then be sent home with prednisone or prednisolone tablets to use over the expected duration of the problem. During the last week or so of this time frame, the dosage would be reduced so the animal is slowly weaned off the medication.

Topical treatments are also very common in veterinary medicine. Many of the topical preparations contain steroids for two purposes. Not only do they help reduce the inflammation present but they also quickly eliminate pain and itching. If we can get the animal to leave the affected tissue alone, it will usually heal much quicker. In many cases, the self-inflicted damage done by the dog is greater than that done by the inflammation. Most medications for ear infections or skin sores utilize steroids for these reasons. Many will contain hydrocortisone, which is rarely used except in topical preparations. Many are produced in combination with antibacterial or antifungal medications. Examples of these would be Panolog, Betasone Topical, and Otomax.

Old dogs commonly have arthritis, a condition made worse by inflammation secondary to abnormal and disfiguring bone changes. Steroids can be and commonly are used in these older patients. They decrease the pain and, if used correctly, have little effect on the rest of the body. Other medications may be utilized first but if these fail or are no longer effective after a period, then steroids can be used. When used for long periods of time, it is still better to try every-other-day therapy. These medications are powerful painkillers for these patients and often allow such animals to live much longer and more comfortable lives. Some anti-arthritic preparations are a combination of methylprednisolone and aspirin. An example of this would be Cortaba.

Autoimmune diseases were mentioned earlier. Steroids are really the only treatment for these potentially fatal diseases. Examples would be **autoimmune hemolytic anemia, lupus, von Willebrand's disease,** etc. Tablet forms of prednisone or prednisolone are again used on an every-other-day schedule. These animals are frequently on medications for life and it is important that the adrenal glands are not adversely affected.

SUMMARY

These are just a few of the thousands of legitimate steroid uses in the dog. They can be abused just like any other medication with doses that are too high, last for too long, or are used in situations where they will do more harm than good. They are sometimes used without a diagnosis, hoping that their euphoric effects will make the animal feel better for a few days. By then, whatever was bothering it will have passed and the case will be classified as a successful cure. With rare exceptions, steroids should only be used when the diagnosis is known and their effects on the case understood.

The glucocorticoids can be a veterinarian's and dog's best friend when the latter suffers from some form of inflammation or autoimmune disease, or is in need of stimulation to return to normal eating and behavior. They can also be an enemy if abused.

The anabolic steroids are usually used only in life-threatening situations. They fill a void, as no other medication can provide their potential benefits. However, their affects vary greatly from case to case and sometimes the hoped-for level of benefit is never realized.

C H A P T E R 1 1

Nonsteroidal Anti-Inflammatory Medications (NSAIDS)

Many of these products are familiar household names. They were developed for use in humans and have a long history of safety. Because of this, some of the products in this category are sold without a prescription and found in numerous over-the-counter brand name and generic forms. They include **acetylsalicylate** (aspirin), **phenylbutazone** (Butazolidin), **flunixin** (Banamine), **acetaminophen** (Tylenol), **ibuprofen** (Advil), **dipyrone** (Novin), and **meclofenamic acid** (Arquel). While all of these have been used for dogs at one time or another, some are known to produce serious side effects without any real advantage.

These medications are excellent anti-inflammatories and painkillers, and some have the ability to lower fevers. In other words, they work on the local level at the site of inflammation by reducing swelling and irritation, plus lessening discomfort by acting directly on the central nervous system. No single medication does all these things equally well, but rather each has certain strong points or advantages. There is no single medication in this group that will function equally well on every dog. To attain the best results, veterinarians often must experiment with several different products to determine which one works best on the individual patient.

In canine medicine, **nonsteroidal anti-inflammatory drugs** are routinely used for the treatment of chronic arthritic or inflammatory conditions, for relief from pain following trauma or surgery, or to combat fevers resulting from infections, surgery, or trauma. *They are sometimes combined with antihistamines or steroids as their effect can be*

103

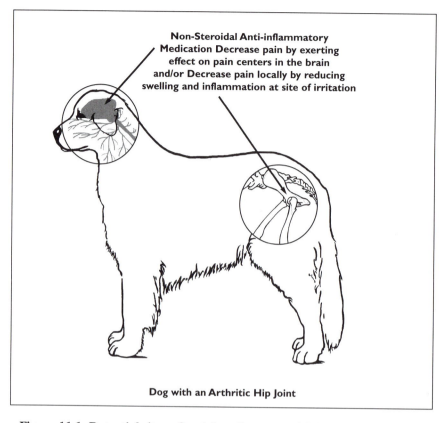

Non-Steroidal Anti-inflammatory Medication Decrease pain by exerting effect on pain centers in the brain and/or Decrease pain locally by reducing swelling and inflammation at site of irritation

Dog with an Arthritic Hip Joint

Figure 11-1: Potential sites of activity of non-steroidal anti-inflammatory products (on irritations such as arthritis).

additive. Under the direction of a veterinarian, different nonsteroidal anti-inflammatories are sometimes used simultaneously with an improved or additive effect.

Acetylsalicylate

Aspirin (acetylsalicylate) is by far the most widely used nonsteroidal anti-inflammatory in canine medicine. It comes in a wide range of orally administered and topical products sold under many brand name or generic labels. It is an excellent product for long or short term therapy for the treatment of arthritis, soft tissue inflammation, fevers, and pain.

Many dogs suffering from disorders such as hip dysplasia easily tolerate acetylsalicylate usage for years. The typical aspirin form so commonly used in human medicine can be used in dogs, but the enteric coated or buffered products (Bufferin or Ascriptin) are *preferred*. Many dogs will have problems with vomiting and diarrhea or bleeding disorders from the *typical* aspirin form. It is therefore recommended that the coated or buffered form be used in canine medicine, as problems are rarely noted even with long term therapy. The potential for side effects with either form is greatly reduced if the product is given with food.

Salicylic Acid

This product is closely related to aspirin, but is generally found in topical preparations. It exhibits the same local anti-inflammatory effects of relieving pain and itching. The product is very safe and moderately effective. It is found in many over-the-counter products such as creams, lotions, and shampoos, and is usually combined with other medications.

Ibuprofen

Sold as a generic or under such brand names as Advil or Motrin, this product can be used for the same conditions as aspirin products. It is also given orally. *In canine medicine, it is more likely to cause gastrointestinal upsets, often with bleeding.* Because of this, ibuprofen is rarely the first choice, especially if long term therapy is planned.

Acetaminophen

Oral forms of **acetaminophen** can be found under numerous generic labels. It is commonly sold under the brand name Tylenol. In dogs, the authors have found it to be useful in cases involving soft tissue pain or fevers, but not very effective in the treatment of arthritis. Some dogs will experience mild gastrointestinal upsets such as vomiting or diarrhea, but bleeding disorders are very rare. Most veterinarians would prefer to use an enteric coated or buffered aspirin product.

Phenylbutazone

Phenylbutazone is a very potent anti-inflammatory available in orally administered or injectable forms. There are numerous generic formulations of this product and it is also sold under the brand name Butazolidine. It is used extensively in the treatment of arthritis and soft tissue swelling and inflammation. In some patients it does a much better job of controlling the pain and discomfort associated with arthritis than other products in this class. Additionally, it is used in the treatment of inflammatory processes that occur inside the eyeball because of its ability to permeate the structure.

As is true with several medications in this class, gastrointestinal upsets such as vomiting and diarrhea are fairly common. Administration with food greatly reduces the incidence of these signs.

More significantly, however, *blood cell abnormalities are also noted.* Phenylbutazone can drastically *suppress* the number of **platelets,** which are responsible for the clotting mechanism of blood, thereby leading to *bleeding disorders.* It can also *prevent the production and release of new red blood cells* into circulation, causing *severe anemias.* Because of these potential side effects, the use of this product must be monitored closely.

In the authors' experience, most dogs tolerate the product without any adverse reactions. Other animals seem to have a predisposed sensitivity to it and problems occur.

Flunixin

Flunixin (Banamine) is a prescription product available in granules that are mixed with food, and also in an injectable form. It is probably a stronger pain reliever than most medications in this class. Uses include treatment of arthritic disorders, soft tissue injuries, and inflammations (including those of the eye). Dogs that have trouble tolerating this product will initially vomit, salivate excessively, and/or have rapid shallow respiration. If these signs are observed, the drug should be discontinued. In some animals the product is **nephrotoxic**—poisonous to the cells of the kidneys—or may cause some ulcerations of the gastrointestinal tract.

Use of flunixin in the dog should be closely monitored by a veterinarian and any side effects should be immediately reported by the owner. In veterinary medicine, flunixin is only approved for use in horses. Veterinarians do, however, use the product in dogs.

Meclofenamic Acid

Meclofenamic acid (Arquel) is closely related to aspirin chemically and has similar actions in dogs. It is given orally, being produced both in granules for horses and tablets for dogs. It is usually used in the treatment of arthritis or soft tissue inflammation. Vomiting, diarrhea, and ulceration of the gastrointestinal tract can occur with its use in the dog.

Dipyrone

Dipyrone (Novin) is available in both injectable and oral forms. Although it has many of the same anti-inflammatory and pain-killing abilities as the other nonsteroidal medications in this group of drugs, it is most commonly used in the injectable form to lower fevers. It is often used in cases of heat prostration in the dog. Although still used in some clinics, this product is no longer manufactured.

Polysulfated Glycosaminoglycan

This equine injectable (Adequan IM) is sometimes used in dogs. Injections are given once every four days, for twenty-eight days. It's usually reserved for severe cases of joint disease or arthritis that do not respond to other approved medications. It may cause bleeding problems and also affect prostaglandin synthesis.

SUMMARY

This class of medications is, in most instances, easy to obtain. They are sold in many over-the-counter formulations that are relatively safe. If the owner of a dog decides to use any of these products, they must do so carefully and be observant for any adverse reactions. The fact that most are safe and can be purchased without a prescription does not mean that higher than recommended dosages should be used without a veterinarian's approval.

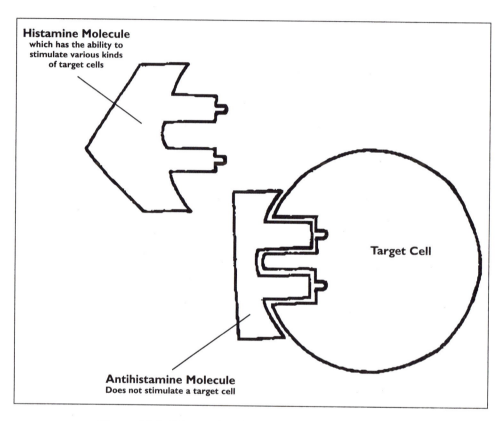

Histamine Molecule
which has the ability to
stimulate various kinds
of target cells

Target Cell

Antihistamine Molecule
Does not stimulate a target cell

Figure 12-1: Schematic of antihistamine vs. histamine.

C H A P T E R   1 2
Antihistamines

Histamine is a substance stored in the body's **mast cells, basophils, and platelets. Mast cells** are found throughout the body within connective tissue. **Basophils** are one type of white blood cell carried throughout the body by the circulatory system. They have the ability to pass from the capillaries into the surrounding tissue. **Platelets** are tiny blood cells responsible for blood clotting following injury or surgery.

Histamine is released from these cells when triggered by trauma, invasion by foreign organisms or cells, inflammation, etc. It is believed that it functions to protect the body by promoting healing through increased cellular activity during these occurrences. In normal, healthy animals this can be very beneficial. However, in some instances, animals develop diseases that alter the activity of their bodies outside of the normal range.

An example would be when hypersensitivity reactions occur or allergies develop. During these occurrences, the body reacts against itself in a way that is far from natural. Normal, healthy animals do not have allergies or develop hypersensitivity reactions. These are reactions against products that are generally not dangerous to the body. However, the immune system sees the initiators of these reactions as foreign or potentially harmful. Histamine causes dilation of the small blood vessels, itching, fluid discharge by cells, and/or swelling of the tissues in the area of its release. Severe generalized reactions often involve the small airways within the lungs. Histamine causes them to constrict, making breathing more difficult.

People and dogs commonly develop simple allergies to pollen. In people it's called "hay fever," while in dogs it is a form of **atopy.** A person develops runny eyes and a stuffed-up nose; the dog suffers from an intense, itchy skin disease. The dog reacts by scratching and chewing to the point of self-mutilation. Both of these disorders are caused by histamine release and its effect on the body's tissues. It is not normal or beneficial but rather a normally functioning protective system that turns against the individual it is intended to protect.

The main role for antihistamines in canine medicine is to counter the effects of the body's naturally produced and released histamine. Specifically this is done in cases involving allergies or similar sensitivity reactions. Those commonly used are **hydroxyzine** (Atarax), **chlorpheniramine** (Chlor-Trimeton), **diphenhydramine** (Benadryl), **terfenadine** (Seldane), and **trimeprazine** (Temaril). Some of these, such as diphenhydramine and chlorpheniramine, are available in over-the-counter formulations while the others are generally by prescription only. They are produced in tablet, capsule, topical, and injectable forms by themselves or in a wide range of combination products that often contain an antihistamine and other anti-inflammatory agents, such as one of the steroids. Most antihistamines are well absorbed after oral administration and carried throughout the body by the circulatory system. Some easily cross the "blood-brain barrier," making their way into the central nervous system.

The mechanism of action of antihistamines is very simple. They are *antagonists* to histamine. They do not alter its production or its release. Rather, they block its attachment to target cells by their physical presence. They simply take the place of the histamine molecules. Because of this, they must be given frequently to be effective. Histamine is constantly being liberated by the mast cells and basophils when allergenic reactions occur. The antihistamines must reach the receptor sites on the target cells before the histamine molecules do. As they break down or are released, a fresh supply must be immediately present or the histamine will make contact with the cells and initiate the unwanted response.

It is obvious that in this type of dynamic relationship between two different and competing molecules, neither will be completely effective. And so it is with antihistamine therapy. It can be very useful but rarely totally eliminates the problem. Dogs suffering from itchy skin diseases brought on by allergies can be helped with antihistamine therapy, but rarely, except in mild cases, can the clinical signs be completely eliminated. When used with other types of medications such as steroids, the antihistamines may significantly lower the amount of steroids needed in the treatment of the disease.

Antihistamine therapy is very safe and serious side effects are rarely observed. At typical dosage levels, the most common sign is sedation or drowsiness. At higher dosages or in animals with extreme sensitivities to these products, gastrointestinal signs such as vomiting or diarrhea may be noted. Some animals will become excited, and in rare cases at very high usage levels, this may extend into seizures. *Antihistamines should not be used in pregnant animals, as deformities have been recorded in the unborn.*

Antihistamines can also be useful in respiratory disorders other than those caused by allergies. These medications suppress the activity of the cough center that is found within the brain. Additionally, they decrease the excessive secretions commonly noted with respiratory infections and inflammations. Most over-the-counter human cold medications contain at least one antihistamine.

The antihistamine **dimenhydrinate** (Dramamine) is used to prevent motion sickness in dogs during travel in vehicles or planes. It prevents vomiting and other signs often associated with motion sickness by suppressing the vestibular apparatus. This structure is found within the inner ear and is important in the maintenance of balance and the awareness of movement.

Cimetidine (Tagamet) and **ranitidine** (Zantac), both antihistamines, are sometimes used in gastrointestinal disorders as they decrease acid production by the stomach wall. This is useful in patients with gastric ulcers. These have also been used successfully in dogs that chronically vomit food or a bile-tinged phlegm. These do not cross the "blood-brain barrier" and therefore do not produce sedation, as is seen with the previously mentioned antihistamines.

PART III

The Pharmacotherapeutic Drugs—The Body Modifiers

The chemotherapeutic drugs work to protect the body from disease-causing organisms or cells of the body that are dangerous to its existence. They don't just build a wall between the patient and these invading disease-causing organisms or cancer cells; rather, these medications actually direct their activity at them. They are the "body defenders."

There are times and medical conditions, however, when the body or its various systems fail to function correctly. Organs or entire systems can be abnormally formed, wear out, or be diseased and unable to do their intended task. In these situations the body's own activity can become just as dangerous to its long-term existence. In these patients, **pharmacotherapeutic agents** are used in an attempt to alter or correct the way the systems function. These medications are referred to as the "body modifiers."

Pharmacotherapeutic medications are used routinely in canine medicine. They exert their activity toward the body's cells or functions, trying to modify them so they remain within a more normal range. These can be given in a single administration, over a brief period of time, or for the life of the animal. Common examples would be an antidiarrheal medication to reduce the motility of the gut in a dog with an irritated gastrointestinal tract; steroids to control an allergy; or an oxytocin injection given to a female in labor to strengthen her contractions.

Medications in this category are not magic. Their use must be closely supervised. If they can alter the function of a system to bring the level of its activity back within the normal range, then an overdose can easily cause an overcorrection. When using any of these medications, the owner is always responsible for informing the veterinarian of any abnormalities or adverse reactions. They will frequently occur. Even animals that are on the same medication for a long period of time may need an alteration in the dosage. Sometimes they may fail to tolerate the product and need to be switched to an entirely different one. It helps if the owner understands what the medication is doing, how it functions, how it can interact with other medicines, and what side effects can occur. This allows the owner to be part of a team in the treatment of his dog.

CHAPTER 13

The Gastrointestinal Tract

The canine gastrointestinal tract is best described as a series of tubes and bags used to store and transport food from the mouth to the anus (see Figure 13-1). While transported, food is subjected to a series of events that change its consistency, allowing nutrients to be extracted and used as fuel by the body's cells. This processing and conversion of food to usable nutrients is known as **digestion.** Each portion of the gastrointestinal tract plays a specific role in the digestive process.

In the mouth, food is chewed and pulverized to break it down. The **esophagus** is a muscular tube which transports food from the mouth to the **stomach.** The stomach is a bag-like unit which temporarily stores food and then slowly releases it into the small intestine. The stomach churns the food and adds stomach acids to aid in digestion. From the stomach, food enters into the **small intestines,** which are several feet in length. Digestive enzymes from the **pancreas** and **liver** are also deposited into the small intestine to be mixed with the food. Absorption of nutrients into the blood system occurs through the wall of the small intestine. The small intestines continuously churn and move the food toward the **large intestine** with wavelike contractions of muscles. The large intestine or **colon** is at the end of the digestive tract. It is here that water is absorbed into the bloodstream and the feces (stool) becomes firm and compacted, ready for elimination from the body.

Many diseases including infections, inflammations, nervousness, motion sickness, and poor enzyme production can upset the digestive system. Various signs can be associated with a malfunctioning digestive tract including vomiting, diarrhea, and constipation.

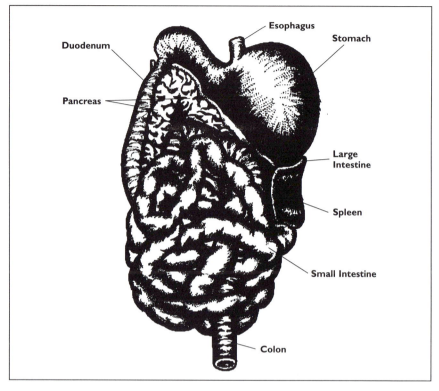

Figure 13-1: Gastrointestinal tract.

These symptoms commonly require treatment involving the usage of specialized drugs to correct the disorder.

ANTIVOMITING PRODUCTS (ANTIEMETICS)

Vomiting is a common sign associated with an upset or irritable stomach. Many things can cause vomiting, including infections, poisons, motion (carsickness), ulcers, nervousness, and parasites.

Vomiting is the expulsion of food once it reaches the stomach. It is possible to vomit on an empty stomach, in which case the vomitus is usually yellow and/or foamy in appearance. A patient that persistently vomits is unable to eat and may actually lose excess fluid, becoming dehydrated. Many drugs are used to stop vomiting in the canine and the selection is often based on the suspected cause. Listed below are some of the more common antivomiting medications prescribed by veterinarians.

Aminopentamide

Once administered, **aminopentamide** (Centrine) slows the rate of contractions of the stomach muscles and therefore acts as an anti-spasmatic. Additionally, it decreases the production of stomach secretions. Side effects can include dry mouth and eyes and an increased heart rate. Centrine will also help prevent diarrhea as it slows intestinal motility. It is available in injectable or in tablet form. *It should not be used in dogs suffering from glaucoma.*

Prochlorperazine

Prochlorperazine (Compazine) is an excellent antiemetic. Prochlor-perazine is also combined with isopropamide and is generally prescribed under the name Darbazine. Darbazine is usually pre-scribed to slow the mobility of the gastrointestinal tract. It can be used to prevent vomiting and/or diarrhea and helps in avoiding motion sickness. Adverse reactions include dry mouth, constipa-tion, and dilated pupils. *Atropine is the antidote if side effects occur. As with Centrine, it should not be used in dogs suffering from glaucoma.*

Metoclopramide

Sold under the brand name Reglan, **metoclopramide** is a drug gen-erally utilized specifically for vomiting. Its principal action is on the stomach and esophagus. *It should not be used in patients with a known history of seizures.*

Dimenhydrinate

The main use of **dimenhydrinate** (Dramamine) is to prevent vomit-ing associated with motion sickness. Motion sickness is typically associated with automobile, aircraft, or watercraft rides. As a side effect, some patients may exhibit a dry mouth due to an inhibition of saliva production. Refer to chapter 12 for a more complete dis-cussion of this medication.

GASTRIC ULCERS

As in humans, some canine patients experience **gastric ulcers.** A gastric ulcer is best defined as an area within the stomach lining that is irritated and inflamed. Ulcers may be as small as the head of a pin or as large as a half dollar. Large ulcers form craterlike pits, eroding through the stomach lining and occasionally through the entire stomach wall as well. The stomach normally produces acids to aid in digestion. Nervousness, stress, and other conditions that cause hypermotility of the stomach may contribute to ulcer formation. An overproduction of stomach acids may also be irritating to the stomach lining and contribute to ulcer formation. The signs of gastric ulcers may be nonexistent in mild cases or more pronounced in severe instances.

Continuous or intermittent vomiting with or without blood or a dark tarry stool can be indicative of gastric ulceration.

Cimetidine

Sold under the brand name Tagamet, **cimetidine** is an over-the-counter, nonprescription drug used to reduce the production of gastric acids. It may be used alone or in conjunction with antacids such as DiGel or Maalox. Side effects are rare, but *the drug should not be used in patients suffering from a disease of the kidneys and/or liver.* In some dogs, both this medication and ranitidine have been successfully used with chronic nonspecific vomiting. These animals would occasionally, over long periods, vomit a clear, bile-tinged, or bloody phlegm.

Ranitidine

Ranitidine (Zantac) is one of the most potent drugs available to decrease gastric acid secretion, at which it is very effective. It is used for the same reasons as cimetidine. Side effects are rare in the canine.

ANTACIDS

Aluminum hydroxide (Rolaids), **calcium carbonate** (Tums), and **aluminum and magnesium combinations** (Maalox and DiGel) are all referred to as **antacids.** They tend to reduce the amount of gastric acid and inhibit the effects of stomach enzymes. **Pepsin,** a powerful enzyme to digest food, also has a corrosive effect and contributes to ulcerations. Antacids will inhibit the enzymatic action of pepsin. Side effects may include constipation.

SURFACTANTS OR ANTIBLOAT AGENTS

Bloat is a true emergency too frequently suffered by many dogs. It was previously thought to occur only in large, deep-chested breeds. Today it is known that it can occur in any dog. After eating, and possibly following exercise, large quantities of gas will be formed in the stomach. A thick, sticky mixture of food and foam will form. The dog is unable to belch up the gas from this mixture because of its consistency. Surfactants are used to eliminate the surface tension within the foam, which allows all of the gas to be freed from the mixture. If this is done early in the condition, surgery may be avoided. Additionally, in animals that have a history of bloat, veterinarians often recommend that their clients give surfactant tablets with every meal for the remainder of the dog's life. This usually prevents bloat-causing foam to form again. Gas is still produced with the food but, in a free form, is easily belched up by the dog.

One of the most commonly used surfactants is **simethicone.** It is found in many generic forms and is also one of the ingredients in DiGel.

ANTIDIARRHEALS

Diarrhea is best described as a frequent discharge of fluid feces from the large bowel. The fecal amount may increase or decrease depending on the amount of food within the bowel. Therefore, diarrhea is not more feces but rather an increased frequency of bowel movements. Diarrhea is usually the result of either an abnormal hypermotility of the intestines or a lack of digestion and absorption of food. Drugs used to treat diarrhea usually lessen the intestinal motility and/or coat the intestines. Generally, if infections are the cause of diarrhea, the coating agents are selected over motility-altering drugs. The increased motility does help expel infectious organisms from the body despite causing diarrhea.

Diphenoxylate
Usually sold under the name Lomotil, **diphenoxylate** is commonly prescribed to aid in the treatment of diarrhea. It works by decreasing the mobility of the intestine. Additionally, it helps control abdominal pain and intestinal spasms. Side effects include constipation and sedation. Lomotil is usually not utilized for more than forty-eight hours.

Bismuth Subcarbonate and Activated Attapulgite
These two substances are combined with **kanamycin** in the brand name Amforol, labeled and approved for use in dogs. They are

antidiarrheal, while kanamycin is an aminoglycoside antibiotic that is not absorbed after oral administration. Amforol is given orally in liquid or tablet form. Side effects (which are very rare) include lethargy, muscle twitching, and seizures. In some dogs, the tongue and stool may be darkened. This is a very popular product.

Methscopolamine Bromide
This medication is found in several generics and in Neosorb-M tablets. It functions by decreasing the motility of the intestinal tract. It also decreases abdominal pain and intestinal spasms. It may lead to constipation and drowsiness in more sensitive dogs or at excessive doses.

Kaopectate
Kaopectate is actually a formulation of **kaolin** and **pectin.** Its main function is to act as an intestinal coating agent. By coating the inflamed intestinal surface it helps improve fecal consistency. Very few side effects are seen; however, with prolonged usage it can cause constipation.

Pepto-Bismol
Pepto-Bismol is a formulation of **bismuth.** Its primary function is to slow the motility of the intestines and soothe any inflammation. Additionally, a protective coating is added to the intestinal wall. Very few side effects are noted; however, constipation may occur. Stools may take on a dark or greenish color.

CONSTIPATION

Constipation is best described as a slower than normal rate of food movement through the gastrointestinal tract. The feces are abnormally firm, even hard. Passing of feces may be painful and difficult. In severe cases, the colon becomes impacted with feces to the point of inability to defecate. The causes of constipation may be any of the following: infections causing a lack of intestinal motility; a lack of adequate fluid intake, resulting in dehydration; abnormal diets or those containing a large quantity of indigestible matter; and loss or interruption of normal nerve supply to the intestine, which prevents normal motility. The ingestion of bones, sand, wood, and the like are the most frequent causes of constipation in the dog.

Petrolatum

Found in a wide range of laxative preparations and sold under the brand name Vaseline, many veterinarians like to flavor this product and give it orally as a treatment for constipation. It lubricates the intestines and their contents, and because of its viscosity, it also draws moisture into the large intestine. It is easier to administer than mineral oil, with much less chance of inhalation into the lungs.

Mineral Oil

Mineral oil is commonly administered orally to help lubricate the intestinal tract. To relieve constipation, mineral oil must pass to the level of the colon. Once ingested, this may take six hours or more. Mineral oil helps coat the bowel and inhibit water absorption, thus keeping water in the feces to promote softness. Only food grade mineral oil should be used. It is important to be very careful when giving this product by mouth; it can easily pass into the trachea and lungs, leading to an inhalation pneumonia. Because of this, many veterinarians and breeders prefer to use flavored petrolatum instead of mineral oil. Additionally, some patients will occasionally vomit the mineral oil, making its usage ineffective.

Psyllium Hydrophilic Mucilloid

This is found under many generic brands but is more commonly known as Metamucil. This is occasionally administered by mouth to help relieve or prevent constipation. It can be mixed with water but is usually mixed with food for dogs. Once ingested, it may take up to twenty-four hours to provide a therapeutic effect. Its principal function is to provide fiber and draw water into the feces to help soften the stool. Although uncommon, it may cause temporary abnormal pain and gas formation. It can be used in the diet for long term therapy and is very useful in dogs with chronic constipation problems.

Glycerin Suppositories

These suppositories are placed into the rectum through the anus. They lubricate the stools but also cause water to be drawn into the colon. This further helps to lubricate the stool and also add bulk. These are very useful in puppies and smaller breeds.

ENEMAS

Enemas are fluid preparations administered through the anus. Warm water can be used, but commercially prepared phosphate enemas are generally utilized. One such enema is the Fleet phosphate enema. Once administered, the enema solutions help soften and lubricate the stools. Additionally, the fluid bulk stimulates a bowel movement. Side effects may include seizures, vomiting, bloody diarrhea, and stupor. These effects are not common, but it should be noted that small dogs (weighing less than ten pounds) and cats should not be administered phosphate enemas. Cats especially show an extreme sensitivity to phosphate solutions.

COLITIS

Colitis is a term used to describe an inflammation of the colon. There are many causes, including infections, autoimmune disorders, and parasites. In many instances the exact cause is unknown. The signs associated with colitis are mucus-covered stools, often flecked with blood. Diarrhea or a softer than normal bowel is usually seen. Because of the irritation, bowel movements may be painful and more frequent than normal. Drug therapy is selected based on the exact cause. Most commonly a chronic colitis of undetermined cause is encountered.

Sulfasalazine

Most commonly, especially in colitis of an unknown origin, **sulfasalazine** (Azulfidine) is selected as the drug of choice for management. Sulfasalazine is administered orally and affects the colon in several ways. It has anti-inflammatory properties in addition to suppressing the immune system. This works especially well in cases where an autoimmune disorder is suspected. It also has antibacterial effects. Occasionally, a patient may exhibit a sensitivity to sulfa-based drugs and one may notice vomiting, diarrhea, fever, and an itching sensation of the skin.

PANCREATIC EXOCRINE INSUFFICIENCY

The **pancreas** is a multi-functioning organ and produces hormones as well as digestive enzymes. The **endocrine** portion of the pancreas produces the hormone insulin while the **exocrine** cells provide the digestive enzymes. If the pancreas fails to provide the proper amounts of enzymes needed for digestion, the patient is suffering from a **pancreatic exocrine insufficiency.** The result is diarrhea, loss of nutrients, and weight loss. Often the stool appears soft, greasy, clay-colored, and in larger than expected quantities. Middle-aged dogs are most likely to be affected. The cause is unknown. Various medications are utilized to replace the needed digestive enzymes.

Viokase-V and Pancrezyme

Viokase-V and Pancrezyme are food supplements containing the enzymes lipase, protease, and amylase. They are formed from pancreases harvested in packing plants, ground up, and desiccated. The enzymes help digest fats, proteins, and carbohydrates. They are supplied in both tablet and powdered forms. In most patients the powder performs better than the tablets. These digestive enzymes are mixed with the food prior to feeding and help in the digestive process. These products simply replace those enzymes not provided by the failing pancreatic cells. The food is "digested," or broken down before it is even eaten, to a point that it can be absorbed by the intestines even before it is eaten. Side effects are few, but abdominal cramping is occasionally noted. The major drawback associated with Viokase-V and Pancrezyme is the expense. *A thorough understanding of cost should be reached between the prescribing veterinarian and the pet owner because affected dogs will need to be on these medications for the remainder of their lives.*

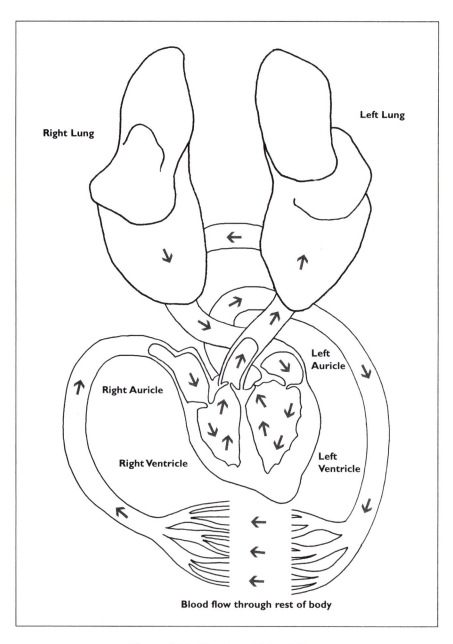

Figure 14-1: Heart and blood flow.

The Heart and Circulatory System

In dogs, as in humans, diseases of the heart are very common. However, the acute heart attack that is so common in people is very rare in dogs. In humans, the blood vessels that supply the muscles of the heart with oxygen and nutrients commonly have materials that build up on the inner walls of those blood vessels. These materials can completely obstruct the vessels, thereby causing areas of the cardiac muscle to function poorly or actually die. If this occurs suddenly, a "heart attack" results.

Dogs rarely suffer from this instantaneous change in the blood flow to the heart. Rather, the common heart conditions develop slowly over a prolonged period of time. Theirs is more of a gradual failure of either valves or muscular walls to function correctly. This often leads to a syndrome we refer to as **congestive heart failure.** Simply stated, this means the heart, which is nothing more than a pump, fails over time.

The other most common cardiac condition in dogs is an abnormality in the rhythm of the contracting or "beating" of the heart. The strong lower chambers (the right and left **ventricles**) beat together, while the upper chambers simultaneously contract a split second later. The actions of these portions of the heart account for the "lub-dub" sounds that we associate with the heart.

These contractions are coordinated by natural pacemakers found within the heart muscles which send out waves of electrical charges, causing the muscles of the various portions of the heart to contract. If these structures are damaged in some way or the muscles cannot correctly receive or pass on these charges, the natural rhythm of the heart's beating is altered. These disorders are referred to as **arrhythmias.** These can be very serious, as they may overwork certain portions of the heart and also prevent the organ from pumping the blood efficiently throughout the animal's body.

The heart is probably the simplest organ in the entire body. With the exception of those needs common to all tissues of the body, it adds or takes nothing from the blood. It is simply a pump responsible for the continuous flow of blood throughout the body.

This blood from the body returns to the right side of the heart. It initially enters the upper *right* chamber or **atrium,** which contracts, forcing the blood through the **right atrioventricular valve** into the lower chamber or **ventricle** on the right side of the heart. From there it is pumped into the lungs, where the blood releases carbon dioxide and gathers oxygen. The right side of the heart is therefore responsible for the oxygenation of the blood. The blood then returns to the **left atrium,** which forces it through the **left atrioventricular,** or **mitral valve,** into the **left ventricle.** This very large, thickly muscled chamber then pumps the blood throughout the entire body. (See Figure 14-1.)

The two common medical disorders of the heart that we mentioned, congestive heart failure and arrhythmia, both affect the ability of the heart to be an effective pump. *Congestive heart failure may be the result of a congenital defect in the heart or it may be acquired as normal cardiac structures age or wear.* They can also be affected by disease or trauma during the life of the dog.

The most common cause of canine congestive heart failure is the *gradual failure of the mitral valve found on the left side of the heart between the atrium and ventricle.* These valves are supposed to close after the ventricle is filled with blood to prevent blood from flowing back into the atrium when the stronger ventricle contracts. In dogs over six years of age, this valve ages and often loses the ability to close completely, allowing some blood to flow back into the atrium during ventricular contraction. (See Figure 14-2.) This overworks the muscular walls of the chambers of the heart as the same blood is pumped over and over in an attempt to move it through the system. The pump starts to fail and each beat of the heart produces inadequate quantities of blood.

Additionally, there are changes in blood pressure in certain areas. Blood starts to build up behind the diseased valve and this becomes especially significant within the lungs, causing blood pressure elevations. In response to this, excess fluid leaves the blood vessels and passes into the tissues of the lungs responsible for carbon dioxide-oxygen exchange. *This prevents the lungs from functioning correctly.* This fluid is commonly referred to as **pulmonary edema** or "fluid in the lungs."

The clinical signs we see with this type of congestive heart failure are *weakness, tiring* with activity, and/or *fainting,* all from inadequate levels of well oxygenated blood reaching the body's tissues. Frequently, the first abnormal sign that owners notice in their pet is chronic coughing as the animal tries to eliminate the fluid within its lungs. Untreated, the condition can be fatal.

With the arrhythmias, the beating of the various heart chambers is not coordinated or properly rhythmic. Each chamber should fill completely and then empty completely with each beat or contraction of the muscular wall. When abnormalities of the heart's natural rhythm occur, a chamber may only be half filled when it contracts or it may wait too long to contract after filling. In either case, this throws the entire system out of coordination as an abnormality in one chamber quickly affects the others. Some chambers will be overworked and finally start to fail.

Simply speaking, arrhythmias or congestive heart failure either prevents the various chambers from filling completely, decreases the ability of the muscle to pump the blood, or both. The end result of either disorder is inadequate profusion of the body's tissues with oxygenated blood, unwanted fluid buildup in certain areas, and failing heart muscle.

The medications used to treat heart disorders in the dog do not cure or eliminate these conditions. Rather, they control them, thereby allowing the heart to work more efficiently. Once the point is reached in the disease that medications are necessary, the patient typically remains on them for the remainder of its life! In fact, in many cases, the medical problem becomes progressively worse; in spite of the therapy, many or all clinical signs remain. However, in most instances the symptoms are eliminated or reduced in severity, and the patient can be maintained in comfort for years. As time passes, a point may be reached when even increased dosages of the medication cannot control the condition, and the patient suffers to some degree. In others, the increased levels of medication needed to control the disease cause harmful side effects that are more severe than those associated with the medical condition. Many of these cases do end with the animal being humanely euthanized.

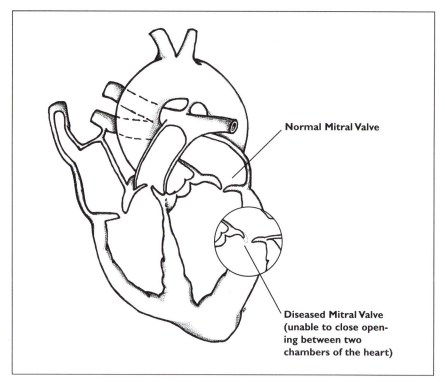

Normal Mitral Valve

Diseased Mitral Valve
(unable to close open-
ing between two
chambers of the heart)

Figure 14-2: Normal and diseased mitral valve.

CONGESTIVE HEART FAILURE

The goal of the medications used to treat this disorder in the dog are to make the heart a stronger, more efficient pump while at the same time reducing the amount of work required of the organ. In some cases, there may be additional medications to deal with problems that are secondary to the failing heart. Remember, none of these products will eliminate or cure the condition. They will only help the heart do its job better while the patient is on the medications. As stated, once therapy becomes necessary it is usually continued for the life of the patient.

In the early stages of congestive heart failure, therapy is generally aimed at reducing the heart's work load. This is done in one of two ways. In one method, it can be accomplished by reducing the amount of fluid that the heart must pump, using medications referred to as **diuretics.** The second method decreases the resistance against which the heart must pump, using **vasodilators.**

Additional medications may also be used that strengthen the heart itself. These compounds work by increasing the ability of the muscles of the heart to contract, thereby increasing force in its pumping actions. Many of these medications also have anti-arrhythmic effects, helping to coordinate the beating of different portions of the heart and allowing the organ to function more effectively.

In many cases of congestive heart failure, diuretics, vasodilators, and those medications that strengthen the heart itself may be used simultaneously or in any combination. The selection of drugs is often refined or altered as their effect on the animal is evaluated. Generally speaking, as the medical condition progresses, the total therapeutic regimen uses increased dosages or additional medications.

DIURETICS

Diuretics simply cause the kidneys to produce higher levels of urine, and in lay terms are often referred to as "water pills." They accomplish this by elevating the amount of ions (such as sodium or potassium) that pass into the urine through the kidneys. As higher levels of these salts pass from the blood into the urine, increased quantities of water are pulled along, thereby lowering the total fluid level within the rest of the body. By decreasing the total fluid volume of the body, these medications decrease the total the work load of the heart. Used correctly, they do not cause dehydration. The patients are allowed to drink the quantity of water they need. What does occur, however, is that the fluids that have accumulated within the lungs or other areas of the body due to the failing heart are picked up by the blood system and excreted by the kidneys. Additionally, the total quantity of fluid within the blood vessels is decreased. As with any pump, a decrease in the volume of fluid that it must move decreases its work load and makes its job easier.

Furosemide

The most commonly used diuretic in dogs with congestive heart failure is **furosemide** (Lasix). This product can be given orally in liquid or tablet forms in the home and is also available in injectable solutions for clinical situations. The dosage varies greatly with the severity of the disease and whether it is used with other medications. Although this is a very safe product that can be used for long periods of time, problems with furosemide use can occur, especially at high dosages.

It can severely depress the levels of sodium and potassium within the body. Lower than normal concentrations of sodium prevent normal kidney function. Not only does this prevent the furosemide from its intended role of decreasing the overall fluid volume of the body, but it also prevents the kidneys from excreting naturally produced toxic wastes from the body. Abnormally low levels of potassium within the body prevent normal muscle contraction. This is life threatening, especially when the muscles of the heart are affected. Dogs with depressed potassium levels can die because their hearts beat too slowly to supply critical areas such as the brain and the heart's own muscle with adequate levels of oxygenated blood. Arrhythmias can also develop in these patients. Additionally, at very high dosages, furosemide can even lead to serious dehydration.

All of these side effects can be eliminated by occasional blood testing to determine the concentrations of the affected electrolytes and the body's overall fluid level. If abnormalities are noted, then the dosage is altered or the patient can be switched to a different medication. In some cases, if only potassium is affected, these deficits can be offset by supplementing increased amounts of this ion with tablets or increased levels in the diet.

Thiazides

A second, less commonly used group of diuretics are the **thiazides.** They also cause the kidneys to alter the levels of sodium and potassium passed in the urine. In so doing, these ions pull higher than normal levels of water from the body into the urine. There are several different compounds in this group and all end with "thiazide" (e.g., **chlorothiazide**). They can also produce side effects by excessively depressing the levels of sodium or potassium within the body but, as with furosemide, this can easily be detected through occasional blood tests. *The thiazides are never utilized in dogs with impaired or diseased kidney function* as they often tend to decrease total blood flow to these organs. It is therefore possible that their use in these animals could further limit the ability of the kidneys to eliminate toxic wastes from the body.

Spironolactone

A final group of diuretics that are sometimes used in canine medicine are those that prevent potassium loss through the kidneys.

These are referred to as the **potassium-sparing diuretics,** and a frequently used example would be **spironolactone** (Aldactone). These are usually not as consistent or as predictable in their results in decreasing overall fluid levels within the body. Prolonged use can cause problems with higher-than-normal levels of potassium within the body.

VASODILATORS

A **vasodilator** is a substance that expands the size of the blood vessels within the body. Vasodilators can affect arteries, veins, or both. By increasing the size of these vessels, there is simply more space to pump the blood. Said another way, the action of these products decreases the patient's blood pressure, thereby making it easier for the heart to pump the blood throughout the body.

There are numerous different vasodilating medications. Some work directly on the blood vessels; others inhibit the actions of naturally occurring substances in the body that work to maintain blood pressure through vascular wall constriction. For the purpose of this book, all of these will be lumped together and their method of action will not be differentiated. Additionally, this discussion will be limited to only the drugs most commonly dispensed for administration by the owner. Injectable products will not be covered here.

In canine medicine, the most popular vasodilating product on the market today is **enalapril** (Enacard). Many veterinarians use this product alone in treatment during the early stages of congestive heart failure. Enalapril functions by decreasing the blood pressure within both arteries and veins. Few side effects are noted with the use of this product. A small portion of animals treated have been reported to show mild gastrointestinal upsets of vomiting or diarrhea. However, many of these have been on several medications simultaneously. Relative to other heart medications, it is very expensive.

Hydralazine (Apresoline) is a vasodilator that works on arteries but not on veins. Additionally, it has been shown that this product works on the heart itself, increasing its output. This a very useful product in canine medicine, especially in conditions affecting the left side of the heart, such as mitral valve failure or insufficiency. *Side effects* can be noted with the use of this product. These include excessive *low blood pressure* (hypotension) resulting in *weakness, lethargy, fainting, and in rare cases even death; gastrointestinal upsets such as vomiting;* and/or *excessive rapid heart rate (tachycardia).* Occasional monitoring by the veterinarian generally prevents any of these from becoming a problem.

CARDIAC STRENGTHENING AGENTS

The hearts of patients suffering from congestive heart failure have reached a point at which they are unable to adequately pump the blood required throughout the body. This means that they are unable to handle all the blood returning through the veins and/or adequately supply the arterial system. Blood may build up in the blood vessels either behind or in front of the heart. The circulatory system is out of balance. Additionally, the blood may not carry adequate amounts of oxygen or nutrients.

Medications that increase the muscular strength of the heart are used to correct this situation. Through controlled stimulation, even the muscles of a failing heart can contract more completely. If you think of the muscles of the heart as those in your arm, these medications directed at the arm would allow you to lift a heavier weight. Additionally, these medications usually slow the heart rate somewhat. This is beneficial, as it allows the chambers to fill more completely before beating (contracting). The heart therefore pumps more blood with each contraction and pumps it with more force.

Many veterinarians prefer to utilize diuretics or vasodilators in the early stages of treatment of congestive heart failure cases, and reserve the cardiac strengthening agents for later in the course of the disease. Most feel that the greatest benefit to the patient comes from the diuretics and vasodilators, as these decrease the work load on the failing heart. Then as the condition progresses and these medications can no longer control the condition, the strengthening agents are used. Each case is different and the response to any medication varies from animal to animal. The total therapeutic regimen utilized on the individual patient may be reached by trying different products and evaluating the animal's response.

Digitalis

Digitalis is the classic cardiac strengthening agent used in veterinary medicine. It comes in two forms, **digitoxin** (Crystodigin) and **digoxin** (Cardoxin or Lanoxin). It is taken in either tablet or liquid form. Digitalis strengthens the failing heart by allowing the muscles of the individual chambers to contract more completely, causing each beat of the heart to move more blood. Additionally, it slows the beating of the heart, permitting the chambers to fill more completely with blood before they contract. This also causes more blood to be expelled with each contraction.

These properties would lead one to believe that the digitalis compounds are the perfect heart medication, but it is effective only within a narrow dosage range. If the amount used is too little, no benefit is derived. If the quantity used is at levels higher than the individual animal can tolerate, potentially harmful side effects often occur. This beneficial dosage range varies greatly from animal to animal and the dog must be closely monitored to achieve the desired results.

Animals that receive dosage levels that are too high for their bodies to tolerate exhibit a wide range of signs. Usually those first noted by the owner are gastrointestinal upsets such as loss of appetite, vomiting, and diarrhea. Life threatening alterations in the heart may be occurring at the same time. Heart rate may be slowed *or* accelerated to dangerous levels; in some patients, arrhythmias may occur. Any of these changes call for an immediate lowering of the dosage or discontinuation of the product completely.

It is usually difficult, if not impossible, to predict which animals will not tolerate digitalis compounds. While most patients receive substantial benefit from them and can be safely and easily treated with these medications, a portion of those with congestive heart failure cannot. It is known that certain conditions may alter the dosage. *Animals suffering from concurrent kidney failure may not tolerate the medication or will at least need lower doses.* The same is true of patients with lower than normal levels of thyroid activity (**hypothyroid**). Low blood potassium that is often seen with the use of certain diuretics may also lower an animal's tolerance of the digitalis compounds. Additionally, *since these products are metabolized within the liver, animals suffering from disease conditions of that organ may not tolerate these medications.*

ARRHYTHMIAS

The normal canine heart has a consistent beating pattern. In the dog, the overall rhythm and rate of the heart's contractions or beats may be altered somewhat by the pressure changes caused by breathing. This is normal.

However, the coordination of contractions between the **upper chambers (atria)** and the **lower chambers (ventricles)** or between the right and left sides of the heart must be maintained if the heart is to work as an effective pump. Each chamber should fill completely before contracting and should be able to empty without excessive resistance. If an individual chamber or side of the heart beats prematurely or hesitates too long to contract, the entire system will be adversely affected. When this happens, an arrhythmia is said to exist.

The rate and rhythm of the heart are controlled predominately by two structures:

1. Nerves traveling between the central nervous system and the heart.
2. The heart's own internal conduction system.
3. There are also compounds circulating through the bloodstream that can affect heart rate, but these are outside of this discussion.

Needs of the body or reactions away from the heart are monitored; to satisfy these, the nerves modify the overall rate of the heart. The actual sequence and timing of the beating of the heart itself are predominately under the control of the heart's conduction system. These natural pacemakers are made up of a series of **nodes** or nerve bundles that pass electrical impulses through the heart muscle to stimulate the coordinated contraction of the various chambers.

The beating of the different chambers is timed such that they are allowed to fill completely before contraction and empty at a time when the area in front of them in the circulatory pathway is prepared to receive that blood. Any deviation from this results in an arrhythmia. Arrhythmias cause the heart to work excessively hard to adequately profuse the tissues with blood. Uncorrected, this leads to cardiac failure and possibly the death of the patient.

Arrhythmias can be brought on by a wide range of disorders; they are not just abnormalities that arise independently within the heart. Many conditions can cause a cardiac arrhythmia. To name a few, they can be the result of imbalances of electrolytes such as potassium, calcium, or sodium; cancer; gastrointestinal upsets; abnormally elevated or lowered body temperature; neural disorders; infections; glandular diseases such as diabetes or hypothyroidism; medications; low blood pressure; etc.

There are numerous drugs used to treat arrhythmias in the dog. They work by altering the effect of nerves upon the heart or by slowing or retarding the heart's internal conduction system. Many times the correct medication and dosage are achieved through trial and error. A medication is chosen and then utilized at an accepted dosage. The patient is then closely monitored to determine the effect.

Digitalis

Either of the **digitalis** compounds, **digoxin** (Lanoxin or Cardoxin) or **digitoxin** (Crystodigin), can be used to treat cardiac arrhythmias. They affect the stimulation of those nerves that arise from the central nervous system and travel to the heart, and they also slow down the activity of the nodes or nerve bundles within the heart. Many of the arrhythmia compounds that are used to treat the atria or upper chambers of the heart are those characterized by excessively rapid heart rates (tachycardia). As mentioned above in the section dealing with congestive heart failure, the digitalis compounds can cause several serious side effects; patients on these medications must be closely monitored. Please review that section for a discussion of these properties.

Quinidine

Quinidine (Quinaglute) is a very old substance used in both human and veterinary medicine. In the treatment of arrhythmias, its action is mostly on the internal conduction system of the heart. It is most useful in the treatment of arrhythmias involving the ventricles or lower chambers of the heart. It slows the passage of contractile impulses across the heart, thereby giving the ventricles time to fill more completely with blood before contracting. It also has a tendency to slightly slow the overall heart rate.

Most side effects noted with quinidine affect the gastrointestinal system, with loss of appetite, vomiting, and diarrhea being those most commonly reported. Some animals will also experience weakness and an excessively slowed heart rate. Quinidine and the digitalis compounds should rarely be used together as quinidine will greatly increase the chances of adverse digitalis side effects.

Procainamide

Procainamide (Procan SR) is a compound closely related to quinidine. Its mechanism of action, effects, potential side effects, and drug interactions are similar. Some patients will experience unwanted side effects from quinidine but not procainamide, or vice versa.

Propranolol

Propranolol (Inderal) is referred to as a beta blocker and is predominately used in cases of arrhythmias involving the atria or upper chambers of the heart. Additionally, there are times that it can be helpful in controlling certain arrhythmias affecting the ventricles or lower chambers of the heart.

Adverse side effects associated with propranolol usage are excessive slowing of the heart rate **(bradycardia),** lowering of blood sugar levels, lowered blood pressure, diarrhea, and breathing difficulties. The effects on the lowering of the patient's blood pressure may be further potentiated if it is used concurrently with diuretics or tranquilizers. *Severe blood pressure drops may be noted in some patients if it is used simultaneously with digitalis compounds.*

SUMMARY

The medications that are used to correct most cardiac problems, and their actions, are very complicated. Additionally, the effect of any medication is very difficult to predict. Over time, dosage and the tolerance of the individual medicine often change in any given patient. Still, these medications usually add considerable time and quality to the life of the affected dog.

CHAPTER 15

The Respiratory System

The respiratory system is composed of the **nasal passages, larynx, trachea** (windpipe), **bronchi** (branches of the trachea entering the lungs), and **lungs.** (See Figure 15-1.)

The canine respiratory system is basically a network of tubes carrying oxygen to the lungs, where it is exchanged for carbon dioxide. The air exchange also provides a regulatory effect on body temperature, as fresh air cools the body.

Although many diseases may affect the lungs and their airways, the end results are airflow blockage due to bronchospasms and/or abnormal fluid accumulated within the lungs themselves (pneumonia). Coughing and difficulty breathing are two signs often associated with problems within the respiratory system. Whether the cause is viral, bacterial, parasitic, allergenic, or traumatic, certain drugs are utilized to better increase ventilation throughout the airways. Additionally, drugs are used to decrease coughing, which is often associated with diseased airways. **Bronchodilators** are drugs used to dilate the airways to facilitate air flow. **Antitussives** are drugs utilized to eliminate or decrease coughing.

Antibiotics and anti-inflammatories such as the corticosteroids are used for similar purposes with problems of the respiratory system as they are in other tissues of the body.

MEDICATIONS TO REDUCE COUGHING
(ANTITUSSIVES)

Butorphanol
Butorphanol is sold under the brand name Torbutrol and is one of the most potent anti-cough medications for use in the canine.

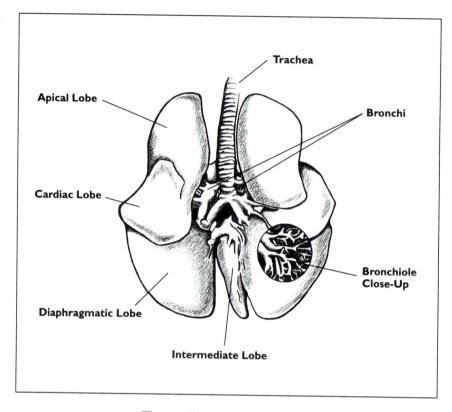

Figure 15-1: Respiratory tree.

Additionally, being a narcotic, it provides pain relief. It is available in both tablet and injectable form; however, the latter is reserved for hospital use only. Side effects include sedation, although usually not marked. Nausea, diarrhea, and vomiting may also be noted. It should not be used in dogs with previous liver disease. How butorphanol functions is not understood but it is believed to act on the cough center of the central nervous system. Since it is so effective, it should not be used in animals with a **productive cough** (coughs bringing up mucus and debris from the chest). This would eliminate the advantageous purpose of coughing.

Hydrocodone (Hycodan)
Hydrocodone is another very potent antitussive and is classified as a narcotic. It may cause sedation, constipation, and vomiting. It is generally prescribed in tablet form but is available as a syrup.

ANTIHISTAMINES (BRONCHODILATORS)

Chapter 12 discusses antihistamines in greater detail. These substances are often used in over-the-counter cough medications, as they also depress the cough center within the brain.

Aminophylline

Aminophylline (Theophylline) is a drug used to dilate the bronchi. Due to irritation, the walls of the bronchi commonly spasm, restricting the openings. Aminophylline reduces bronchospasms, facilitating the passage of air to and from the lungs. *Side effects may include increased urination, diarrhea, vomiting, and poor appetite. It is often used in dogs with heart disease.*

Dextromethorphan

This non-narcotic cough suppressant is found in over-the-counter preparations. It acts on the cough center of the brain but does little to relieve pain or discomfort, unlike butorphanol and hydrocodone.

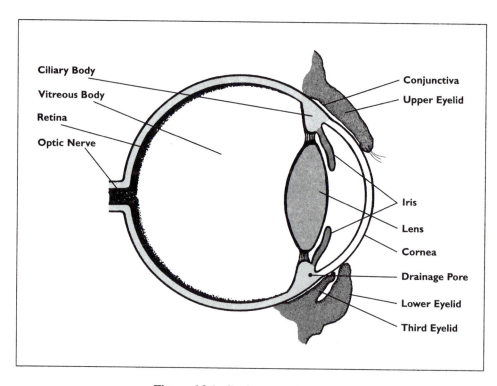

Figure 16-1: Canine eye structure.

CHAPTER 16

The Ophthalmic System

Medical treatment of the eye closely parallels that of other areas of the body; however, there are conditions and therefore medications that are unique to the eye. Antibiotics and anti-inflammatories such as the corticosteroids are used for similar purposes as they are in other tissues of the body. Certain cautions and/or limitations are placed on their use, but the principles are the same. We will limit our discussion to the topical or orally administered products that the owner may be asked to administer and not detail those medications used in a clinic or hospital setting

Ocular problems, when medicated by the owner, are generally treated through topically or orally administered medications. Orally dosed products, with rare exceptions, must follow the same principles as those used to treat other areas of the body. They must be formulated in such a way that the active ingredients will be absorbed by the gastrointestinal tract and then carried by the blood to the target area—in this case, the eyes and their related tissues.

Many eye treatments are administered **topically,** that is, applied directly on the surface of the eye or the surrounding lids. These preparations are formulated in different manners to facilitate their usage. The two most common are ointments and solutions. Ointments come in small tubes and are thick preparations, typically with lanolin or petrolatum jelly as a base. This formula requires less frequent administration, remains in contact with the surface of the eye longer, actually forms a protective film, and softens matter and debris often present in ocular infections or disorders. Solutions, on the other hand, are typically packaged in tiny bottles and applied by letting small drops fall onto the exposed surfaces of the eye. For many owners, solutions are easier to apply and do have an advantage in that they do not cause foreign materials to stick to them as ointments may. Because of their thinner consistency they naturally spread quickly into the tiny recesses and ducts surrounding the eye. They must, however, be applied frequently, usually every one to two hours. Whether a medication is carried in an ointment or a solution has little effect on its absorption into the deeper tissue layers or even the eyeball itself. This is determined by the chemical properties of the compound, not the form in which it is carried.

GENERAL EYE CARE AND THE MEDICATIONS USED

CORTICOSTEROIDS

Corticosteroids in ophthalmic medicine are used as anti-inflammatories. They include **dexamethasone, prednisone, prednisolone,** and **betamethasone.** There are many others but these are the most common. They are found in hundreds of topical preparations or in tablet form.

In addition to their general anti-inflammatory effects, corticosteroids have the ability to eliminate or prevent the formation of blood vessels, cellular infiltrates, white blood cell deposits, and scar formation. These properties are the reason for their use in many diseases of the **cornea,** which is the clear outer membrane covering the surface of the eye. Many diseases such as pannus, or ulcers in this area, require their use at all or certain stages of treatment.

Corticosteroids should never be used during the early stages of a corneal ulcer as they may prevent correct healing and even cause scar tissue to form within the cornea.

It is interesting to note that if the medications are applied topically rather than given orally, they are more effective. Their passage into the eyeball through the bloodstream is very poor.

ANTIMICROBIALS

A wide range of antibiotics is used in the treatment or prevention of ocular infections. To be effective against the typical ocular infection that affects the surface of the eye and lids, they must be administered topically. Topical application also allows the use of compounds that will not be absorbed orally, such as gentamicin. The **sulfonamides** are antimicrobials that are contraindicated in ophthalmic infections or that may need to be avoided for ocular problems. It has been shown that these may cause or predispose a dog to **keratitis sicca** or "**dry eye syndrome.**" After administration, they decrease the quantity of tears produced and in some cases, this may be a long term or lifelong phenomenon.

OPHTHALMIC PAINKILLERS

To examine eyes in a clinic situation, a veterinarian may use a topical painkiller or local anesthetic. These are special products not used by owners at home.

There are times, such as with a severe injury or a corneal ulcer, when dogs may paw or rub their eyes in response to pain even after other topical treatments have been initiated. Veterinarians typically dispense an **atropine solution** for this purpose. Drops are usually only applied for two to three days, as by then the healing eliminates discomfort to the dog. A side effect will be a dilated pupil that may last for a day or two after the atropine drops are discontinued.

SPECIFIC OCULAR DISORDERS IN WHICH MEDICAL THERAPY IS UTILIZED

Although there are numerous diseases and medical conditions that affect the eye, many can be cured or successfully managed using medications alone. Some disorders of the eye are treated surgically, with the follow-up medical therapy being similar to other conditions.

Below we describe two ocular disorders that are both very common and usually require medical therapy utilizing specific and unique products.

KERATOCONJUNCTIVITIS SICCA (KCS)

Dry eye syndrome is also referred to as **keratoconjunctivitis sicca (KCS)**. In this disorder, the **lacrimal** or tear producing glands of the eye fail to function correctly and produce less than the normal quantity of tears. Tears have many functions. Among these, they kill bacteria and lubricate the surfaces of the lids and eyeball while keeping the surface of the cornea moist. Without an adequate covering or film of tears, the cornea dries. If this happens it becomes cloudy, interfering with vision and hardening so that gases such as oxygen can't pass through it into the deeper structures of the eye. The cornea then eventually dies.

This is a painful condition that requires treatment to prevent blindness. The condition often occurs simultaneously in both eyes. Since tears are bactericidal, topical antibiotic preparations are always used in addition to the following preparations.

Artificial Tears

These preparations are placed on the exposed surface of the eye repeatedly throughout the day. Their only purpose is to keep the cornea moist so that it can continue to function as intended. Brand names such as Hypotears, Tears Natural, or Adapt belong to a group with a special ingredient (mucin polyvinylpyrrolidine) that causes the solution to remain on the surface of the eye longer than other solutions. Ointment style artificial tears are also available under such names as Duratears or Tears Renewed. As with all ointments, they require fewer daily applications than solutions.

Products That Stimulate Tear Production

Lacrimomimetic products stimulate increased tear production from the lacrimal (tear) glands. Most dogs with dry eye (KCS) still have *some* functional glandular tissue, but it does not produce adequate quantities of tears.

Cyclosporine

In the last few years cyclosporine (Sandimmune) has been formulated in two-percent solutions that can be applied directly to the surface of the eye. This medication was actually developed as an immunosuppressant for use in autoimmune diseases and this formulation has proven to be an excellent addition to the treatment of dry eye (KCS). A small percentage of animals exhibit signs of irritation or discomfort briefly after its administration.

Pilocarpine

Pilocarpine drops (available in a wide range of generic and brand name products), another tear stimulating (lacrimomimetic) compound, can also be used to treat KCS. These drops can be placed topically into the eye or given orally, often mixed with food. Since the advent of cyclosporine therapy, pilocarpine is less commonly used for KCS. Topical administration of this product causes the pupil to constrict or become smaller. Additionally, it often causes severe ophthalmic irritation. Orally, it can cause gastrointestinal disturbances such as diarrhea, vomiting, loss of appetite, and excessively elevated heart rates. *It should not be used in dogs suffering from most forms of heart disease.*

GLAUCOMA

This disease is one of the most serious ophthalmic conditions affecting dogs. It is characterized by excessively high pressure inside the eyeball. The eyeball produces a liquid referred to as the **aqueous humor** which fills the center of the eyeball, maintaining the eye's shape and supplying oxygen and nutrients to the structures inside the eye. This fluid is produced constantly and therefore, in the normal eye, it must be eliminated constantly.

Glaucoma results whenever fluid produced cannot drain correctly from the eye. **Primary glaucoma** is the result of conformational abnormalities that are genetically transmitted from generation to generation. This hereditary predisposition is much more common in some breeds, but can occur in almost any dog. Many animals that suffer from primary glaucoma will develop the condition in both eyes. **Secondary glaucoma** is the result of infections, trauma, cancer, etc. Both forms are treated similarly.

Glaucoma Treatment
Some form of surgery may be necessary to completely correct the problems associated with glaucoma in the dog. Even if this is done, however, most cases also employ various forms of medical therapy. The absence of treatment almost *always* leads to total blindness.

Medical therapy is directed at the level of fluid in the eye. To decrease the pressure, medications either strive to lower the quantity of liquid being produced or make it easier for the liquid present to more easily drain from the globe. In all but a few cases of secondary glaucoma, the therapy continues for the life of the animal once initiated. A cure is rarely achieved in this extremely painful disorder. Therefore, unless the eyeball is surgically removed, therapy may be continued even after the animal's sight has been lost.

Medications to Increase Fluid Drainage
Pilocarpine
This is the same medication that is used to increase tear production

in dogs suffering from KCS. In the treatment of glaucoma it is administered topically onto the surface of the eye several times a day. As in KCS, its administration is followed by a decrease in the size of the pupil. In some animals, the surface of the eye and surrounding tissues may become inflamed.

Medications That Decrease Fluid Production

Most dogs suffering from glaucoma are placed on these medications. Two commonly used tablet preparations are **dichlorphenamide** (Daranide) and **acetazolamide** (Diamox). Veterinarians may experiment with dosages of these or other oral medications, as individual products may work better with fewer side effects on different animals. Most side effects noted are related to gastrointestinal disturbances such as loss of appetite, vomiting, diarrhea, etc. The overall health of animals on these products is usually monitored through physical examination and blood work to ensure that no additional abnormalities are present.

Topical Medications That Decrease the Production of New Fluid
Epinephrine

This decreases the production of new fluid and to a lesser degree opens up the drainage area, permitting the loss of some existing fluid. It is applied topically onto the eye surface several times daily. It is sold under several trade names including Glaucon and Epifrin. It can't be used on all forms of glaucoma, *nor is it well tolerated by all dogs*. Some dogs experience irritation at the site of administration. Others, after absorption of the product, develop abnormalities such as rapid heart rates, arrhythmias, and elevated blood pressures. It should not be used in animals suffering from concurrent heart disease.

Timolol Maleate

This medication decreases the quantity of the intraocular fluid produced *and* may increase the amount that drains from the eye. Sold under the trade name Timoptic, it comes in a solution that is administered topically onto the eye several times a day. *As with epinephrine, this product should not be used in most patients that are also suffering from heart disease.* Local irritation of the eye may also be noted immediately after use.

CHAPTER 17

The Otic System

Most dog owners, at one time or another, must assist in the treatment of their pet's ears. The active ingredients of the medications used are discussed in other sections of the book, but to be complete, the principles are outlined here.

The most common problem is an infection of the outer ear, i.e., the area outside of the ear drum such as the ear canal. As a matter of fact, after vaccinations and sterilization procedures, this may be the most common reason a dog owner brings an animal to a veterinary clinic. These infections can be caused by bacteria, fungus, yeast, or mites. In some cases, they can come from allergies or infections elsewhere on the body and can have a wide range of environmental causes.

Most preparations are combination products; there are hundreds of them. They all contain something to kill or eliminate the disease-causing organism. This could be an antibiotic, a miticide, or an antifungal. Additionally, these preparations will usually have an anti-inflammatory to reduce inflammation and pain. Most commonly this is a steroid, although a few will use nonsteroidal preparations such as salicylic acid. Some will also contain ingredients that dissolve or break down wax.

These preparations come in liquids, ointments, creams, or sprays. Ointments or creams are usually only applied once or twice daily, while the liquids or sprays may need to be done more often.

Owners should be aware of common mistakes that occur with the use of these products:

- *Treat long enough.* We usually recommend that they be used until the ear canal looks, acts, and smells normal and then

147

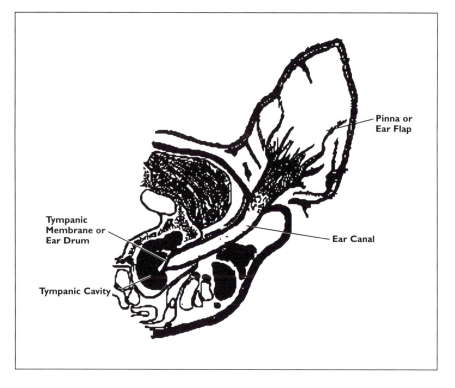

Figure 17-1: Canine ear.

therapy should be continued for an additional four days. If treatment is discontinued too soon, the infection usually returns quickly and may be more difficult to eliminate.

- *Don't use too much medication.* Owners often believe that if one or two drops of a preparation are okay, then ten drops would be even better. This just isn't true. The ear canal needs to be relatively free of material so it can get air. If it is filled with fluid, the problem usually gets worse. It is better to use a small quantity several times a day rather than one large amount.

- *Clean out excess medication* and debris at least once every day or two. If the ear is very painful, this may have to wait for a few days so that the anti-inflammatory portion of the preparation can reduce the swelling and discomfort. This allows the active ingredients a chance to come in contact with the problem-causing organisms and therefore a better chance to eliminate them.

- *Have the animal rechecked* if after five days there seems to be no improvement. A different preparation may be tried or additional tests done.
- *Keep the ear clean* with one of the many solutions formulated for this purpose. After an infection has been eliminated, cleaning eliminates excess wax and debris that unwanted organisms grow on.
- *Keep the ear canal dry.* Try not to get water into the ear canal during bathing. If you do, clean and dry it when you are finished. The same is true for all dogs that swim; dry the ear canals after swimming. Some dogs suffer from chronic outer ear infections, but even in these animals, these simple rules will help to cut down on the frequency and severity of the problems.

Infections and inflammations of the middle and inner ear, i.e., those areas inside of the ear drum, are usually treated with antibiotics and anti-inflammatories. This is done with oral and/or injectable products. These may take longer than would be expected, as it is often difficult to get adequate levels of medication to these areas; furthermore, the structures have no way to naturally drain or expel debris associated with infections.

Ears are treated just like the other areas of the body. There are very, very few medication ingredients that are solely for use on this area.

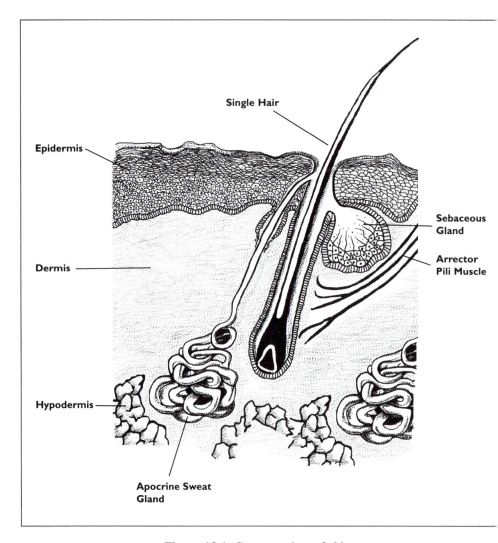

Figure 18-1: Cross-section of skin.

The Skin and Related Structures

When considering treatment of the skin, it is important to understand its anatomy and growth. In the dog, what we see and touch when petting the animal are the most mature cells forming the outer layer of skin. This is true whether we are talking about the hair or the skin itself. The skin, also referred to as the **integumentary system,** is made of numerous layers of **epidermal cells, glands,** and **hair follicles.** Skin develops or matures slowly, with this process starting in the deepest layers. (See Figure 18-1.) The newly formed, most immature epidermal cells are in this lowest area. They are pushed upward by newly forming cells below them. As they move up they mature, harden, and cornify, then finally die. Superficial dead cells may stay attached to and are an important part of the skin, providing protection.

Shampoos and other topical treatments usually only come in contact with and affect the older, more mature cells. Some medications are designed to penetrate to the lower levels but few actually do this. Topically applied products must start from the outer areas and work down into the skin.

When one adds a nutritional supplement or medication to the diet to improve the quality of the skin or hair, the product first reaches the lower layers, enters these cells, and then must be carried up through the various layers until it reaches the surface. This will usually take several days to weeks. When one adds a fatty acid supplement to the diet to add more oils to the skin, it may take three to five weeks before the improvement may be apparent.

SHAMPOOS

Shampoos can be formulated to clean the skin and hair or they may be medicated to deal with a problem. Sometimes the term "medicated" is used in the name of a shampoo when it has no medical formulation or purpose. In these, the use of the term is simply a marketing ploy. Shampoos, whether they are medicated or not, should clean the skin and carry away unwanted materials.

Shampoos may contain soaps or detergents to clean the skin and hair and remove dirt, oil, or other debris. Soaps are a combination of alkali; fats or fatty oils; and salts such as sodium, potassium, or magnesium. Soaps do not function as well in hard water because they leave a residue of salts on the skin and hair. Soaps can be mild or harsh.

Detergents that are used in shampoos are usually synthetic substances referred to as **surfactants.** These break down the surface tension of water so that oils and debris found on the skin and hair can be more easily lifted from the body and rinsed away with water following the bath. Detergents by themselves can be harsh but are often buffered by other ingredients to eliminate these properties. Among the detergents commonly used in dog shampoos are **sodium laureth sulfate, cocamide diethanolamine, cocamidopropyl betaine, disodium cocamphodiacetate,** or **disodium oleamide monoethanolamine sulfosuccinate.**

MEDICATED SHAMPOOS

Medicated shampoos can be antimicrobial, antiseborrheic, or anti-inflammatory. When these products actually have these actions, they are medical products. To call a shampoo "medicated" simply because it sounds good or adds to sales should not be allowed.

Medicated shampoos have a wide range of ingredients in addition to a soap or detergent base. They are often responsible for removing or preventing some problems and they must also be able to clean the skin and coat adequately. Medicated shampoos are usually available over-the-counter. There are a few that are sold by prescription only, but in most cases the same active ingredient at the same concentration can also be found in over-the-counter ones.

Shampoos that are **antimicrobial** may function against *bacteria, fungal organisms, or parasites.* Antibacterial shampoos may contain **benzoyl peroxide** (Vitasheen Benzoyl Peroxide or Oxydex), **chlorhexidine** (Nolvasan), **sulfur** (Lytar or Vitasheen Sulfur-Tar), **iodine** (Betadine), etc. Of these, most veterinarians today prefer those containing benzoyl peroxide, which are very effective against bacteria, but also open up and flush out the hair follicles that contain bacteria. **Antibiotics** are what most people generally perceive as the preferred products against bacterial species, but they are generally not used in shampoos. Rather, for the skin they are applied in creams or ointments. In shampoos they would usually break down quickly or interact with other ingredients. To be truly effective in serious skin infections, oral or injected antibiotics or other antibacterials are usually used concurrently with these medicated antibacterial shampoos.

Antiseborrheic shampoos are used in the treatment of seborrhea. This condition is not always what many dog owners believe it to be. It commonly can be characterized by greasy skin, lots of free dander or scale, and a foul odor. In the mind of most dog owners, these alone are the signs of seborrhea. It can, however, be a very dry, odorless condition that is only associated with scaling and free dander within the coat. Seborrhea is an excess of skin layers. The various layers simply develop or mature too rapidly, with the excess being constantly sloughed off. Sometimes this also affects the oil glands, leading to grease and odor. Antiseborrheic shampoos are responsible for removing excess cells and oils without harming the skin further. Additionally, they must be formulated not to stimulate the skin into further production. Whenever antiseborrheic shampoos are used, they should be left on for several minutes to allow them to completely exert their effect. Additionally, users can be more aggressive with their hands in massaging the coat to break down the excess surface layers.

Antiseborrheic shampoos commonly contain **tar, sulfur, and salicylic acid** (Lytar or Vitasheen Sulfur-Tar) or **benzoyl peroxide** (Vitasheen Benzoyl Peroxide or Oxydex). These products loosen up the excess cells, oil, and debris from the coat and allow them to be removed from the dog's body. Sulfurs found in shampoos are not very good at removing oils and grease but tar improves these qualities somewhat. The sulfur is excellent at removing the upper layers of dead and decaying cells that normally would lift off the surface of the skin to form dander. For this reason, most veterinarians prefer to use them in dry seborrhea.

Salicylic acid (a substance closely related to aspirin) is very useful in relieving the itching and irritation often associated with seborrhea. It does stimulate the production of new epidermal cells but in a very controlled and beneficial manner.

Benzoyl peroxide is excellent at lifting off the older, excess epidermal cells and removing oils and grease. It is so effective at the latter that it should not be used on dry forms of seborrhea, as it may further dry out the skin. Benzoyl peroxide shampoos are always preferred for oily seborrheas.

Anti-inflammatory shampoos relieve inflammation, irritation, and itching. They are a popular treatment for dogs suffering from allergies, hot spots, ectoparasites, or other inflammatory skin diseases. Common examples are those containing **hydrocortisone** (Dermagard or Stop Itch), **oatmeal** (Francodex Oatmeal or Vitasheen Oatmeal), an **antihistamine** (Relief), or **moisturizing agents** (HyLyt *efa). To get the greatest potential from any of the anti-inflammatory shampoos, they must be used often. In severe allergies, hydrocortisone shampoos are very helpful if they are used every two to three days.

Hydrocortisone shampoos have an immediate effect on the skin. They relieve itching, redness, and inflammation. Hydrocortisone is a glucocorticoid and its properties are discussed in chapter 10. Most shampoos are a 0.5 percent concentration. These products are formulated with the understanding that some may be ingested by the dog through licking and some of the product may be absorbed through the skin. Toxicity problems do not occur regardless of the frequency of their usage.

Oatmeal shampoos are excellent cleansing and anti-inflammatory agents. They do an excellent job of soothing irritated skin. They are frequently used in patients with allergies, ectoparasites, and bacterial skin infections. Additionally, many exhibitors use them because their animals must be bathed frequently yet the oatmeal products do not dry out the coat. These individuals also like the body the colloidal oatmeal adds to the coat in long-haired breeds.

Antihistamine shampoos are popular for dogs with allergies. Histamine release is stimulated by the allergen. Antihistamines do not prevent its release but rather block its action by tying up the sites where the histamine would attach and exert its effect. To have any appreciable effect, these products must be used every one to two days or just prior to the animal coming in contact with the allergen. Generally speaking, the antihistamine shampoos should be considered only a small part of the overall therapy of patients suffering from allergies.

MOISTURIZING SHAMPOOS AND AGENTS

Moisturizing shampoos are a treatment for animals with dry skin. They add moisture or increase the quantity of water in the uppermost layers of the skin. Others prevent loss of moisture already within the skin. Various **oils, lanolin,** and **petrolatum** are common ingredients in these mixtures. These are available in a wide range of over-the-counter formulas. Often the moisturizing agent is only one of several ingredients found in the preparation.

RINSES

These liquid products contain therapeutic components that flush through the hair coat, usually after bathing. They can contain antimicrobial, antiparasitics, moisturizers, or any of a wide range of topically applied medications. A common example would be Fungisan, a rinse used in cases of ringworm. The animal is bathed to remove debris and excess oil and then rinsed or soaked with the product over and over to leave an antifungal product within the hair coat.

Whether rinses are purchased with or without a prescription depends on the active ingredients involved. Most common rinses can be purchased over-the-counter.

POWDERS

Most powders applied to the coat of a dog are for the control of ectoparasites such as fleas, mites, or lice. These are covered in chapter 8. There are other powder products used topically on dogs. Among the most common are the "dry shampoos." These attach to oils and debris within the coat and are then simply brushed from the coat. These are useful for animals that will not tolerate bathing with water. They do not clean as well as shampoos used with water but are a popular product with some owners.

OINTMENTS, CREAMS, LOTIONS, AND TOPICAL SPRAYS

There is a wide range of these topical products. Most are mentioned in other chapters of this book dealing with the active ingredients contained within them. Some products are fairly unique in the therapy of the skin and are mentioned below.

Hydrogen Peroxide
This product is available over-the-counter and has strong antibacterial activity—providing the product is in direct contact with the microorganisms for at least a minute or so. Additionally, it breaks down blood, debris, and necrotic material. It is typically used to flush or clean infected areas or cuts and abrasions.

Dimethyl Sulfoxide
Dimethyl sulfoxide is commonly referred to as **DMSO.** It is a liquid sold under generic names and also under the brand names Domoso and Synotic. DMSO is a product seemingly used for almost everything but labeled only for topical use in dogs to remove swelling or relieve itching and inflammation associated with external ear infections.

When applied topically, DMSO has anti-inflammatory effects. More importantly, it rapidly penetrates the skin, entering the dog's bloodstream. It is found at significant concentrations in the various internal organs of the body within minutes. One of its unique properties is that it carries other often unrelated substances with it as it passes through the various skin layers. It can be used to carry antimicrobials, local anesthetics, and other anti-inflammatories into and through the skin.

In humans, DMSO is used to relieve pain, swelling, and itching. It is not just for topical use, but also for internal problems associated with pain and inflammation, such as arthritis and degenerative joint diseases.

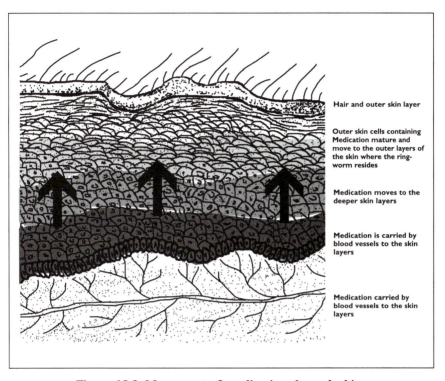

Hair and outer skin layer

Outer skin cells containing Medication mature and move to the outer layers of the skin where the ringworm resides

Medication moves to the deeper skin layers

Medication is carried by blood vessels to the skin layers

Medication carried by blood vessels to the skin layers

Figure 18-2: Movement of medication through skin.

Toxicity problems associated with DMSO are usually not from the product itself but are caused by other substances carried with it.

SUMMARY

There are numerous skin medications covered in other chapters of this book because their active ingredients can be used in many areas of the body.

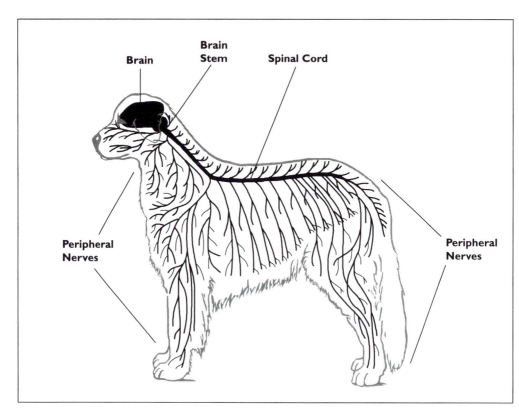

Figure 19-1: Canine nervous system.

CHAPTER 19

The Nervous System

The nervous system is composed of the **central nervous system** (CNS) and the **peripheral nervous system** (PNS). The central portion consists of the brain and brain stem, found within the skull; and the spinal cord, which is encased within the backbone, or vertebrae. (See Figure 19-1.) The peripheral portion is made up of all the nerves that communicate back and forth between the central nervous system and the rest of the body. The central peripheral nerves run directly from the brain to areas of the head and neck, while in the rest of the body, peripheral nerves go back and forth between the spinal cord and all other structures (the abdominal organs, limbs, skin, etc.).

The PNS is the body's mechanism for communicating with the higher centers of the brain and spinal cord. It is divided into motor and sensory nerves. The motor ones, through stimulation initiated within the CNS, bring about movement by the contraction of muscles. The sensory nerves relay information derived from the senses of touch (heat, cold, movement, and pain), hearing, sight, smell, and taste back to the central nervous system.

Numerous medications are used to treat medical disorders of the nervous system, such as damage or inflammation caused by trauma, seizures, and motion sickness. Therapy for these conditions can be done for a brief period following a single incident, for the life of the animal after a problem has developed, or on an "as needed" basis in the case of motion sickness. In most cases, their activity is directed at and has an effect on the central nervous system.

Drug therapy directed at the nervous system is used to facilitate other medical procedures or to calm the animal, as with anesthetics, sedatives, or tranquilizers. With the exception of local or topical anesthetics, all of these medications work on the central nervous system.

MEDICATIONS FOR NERVOUS SYSTEM TRAUMA

Treatment of trauma to the nervous system usually follows injuries to the brain or spinal cord. Such injuries are commonly seen when the dog has been hit by a car, suffered some sort of blow or bite to the head or back, or ruptured a disc between the vertebrae of the back. Such trauma to the central nervous system can result in either destruction of tissue, hemorrhage, or edema. All of these are serious and treatment must be initiated immediately for the best possible prognosis.

In the case of actual destruction of nervous tissue, little can be done as it does not regenerate. The animal will either die or be humanely euthanized if the affected portion is essential for life. In cases in which the destroyed tissue is less critical, the animal must learn to compensate for the loss.

Most traumatic injuries to the nervous system are less severe than this, however, and result in either **hemorrhage** or **edema. Hemorrhage** (bleeding from a vessel) can cause damage in one of two ways. In the first, the vessels that are responsible for carrying oxygen and nutrients to the nervous system are ruptured, with the blood being lost elsewhere. If this is complete, the deprived nervous tissue will die. In the second and more common result of hemorrhage, the blood that is spilling from vessels puts excessive pressure on the nervous tissue.

Edema is the buildup of fluid in or around the nervous tissue. This is the result of bruising or injury to cells that causes them to leak fluid into the area. This can damage and/or affect the ability of nervous tissue to function correctly. A severe sprain of your wrist may cause the area to become swollen, followed by numbness of your hand. A similar reaction can occur anywhere within the CNS or PNS. Nerve cells or fibers are similar to a garden hose in that with severe trauma, you can destroy it, but with pressure alone you prevent it from functioning. Squeeze on it and water will be unable to pass through. The same occurs with nerves. Put pressure on them and the impulses they produce or transmit will not conduct through their fibers.

Since the brain and spinal cord are both encased in bone, there is little if any room for them to enlarge. Both hemorrhage and edema can either take up additional space or actually enlarge the brain and the spinal cord. Since they are confined within bone, their swelling or enlargement causes internal pressure and either the cells are destroyed or neural transmission is impaired. A ruptured disc in the back has the same effect. As it pushes against the spinal cord, it can crush the tissue and destroy it, cause hemorrhage or swelling (edema), or pinch off nerve flow as it extends upward. (See Figure 19-2.) While it is possible sometimes to surgically remove a hemorrhage of free blood or clots, this is rarely practical in veterinary medicine. On the other hand, surgery is frequently done to relieve the pressure caused by a ruptured or herniated disc in the dog. However, in all of these cases, the first and preferred therapy is to use medications to reduce the swelling or pressure brought on by edema, hemorrhage, or a ruptured disc.

Mannitol

In severe cases of trauma through injury or with a ruptured intervertebral disc, hemorrhage or edema may cause a complete or rapid loss of nerve function. The resultant swelling may be so severe that the pressure on the tissue not only prevents any nerve transmission, but can even damage and destroy the nervous tissue.

In these extreme, rapidly deteriorating cases, Mannitol may be used intravenously. Mannitol is a concentrated, sterile sugar solution. Because so much sugar is dissolved in this liquid, it is basically "thicker" than the normal body fluids. Therefore, when Mannitol is given intravenously to one of these patients, it tends to suck the excess fluid from the swollen tissues into the adjacent blood vessels. This causes the tissue and surrounding areas to shrink. As the affected structures decrease in size, the pressure is relieved and the chance of serious or permanent damage decreases. In most cases, the nerve tissue returns to normal function in a short time.

To be effective, Mannitol solutions must be given intravenously and are therefore only used in a hospital situation. They would have no effect if taken orally, and if done subcutaneously, all of their effect would stay where injected.

Mannitol cannot be used when the patient is suffering from shock or has lost large quantities of blood. In those cases the animal is already suffering from inadequate blood or fluid volume within its body's tissues and Mannitol would further complicate these problems.

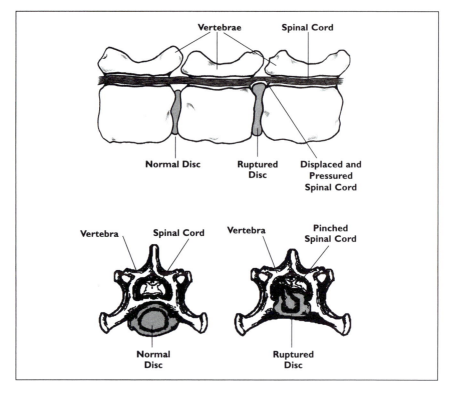

Figure 19-2: Normal and slipped disc.

CORTICOSTEROIDS

In less severe cases of hemorrhage or edema, and particularly in those involving a ruptured intervertebral disc, **corticosteroids** are used. These medications reduce swelling and inflammation from all areas of the body and are very useful in the nervous system. They cause the excess fluid from the swelling to pass into the bloodstream, be carried away from the area, and out through the kidneys. They also act on the *adjacent* disc. Higher doses are typically given for the first day or so and then the dosage is slowly decreased over the next several days or weeks depending on response. Initially this is done by injection, but later oral forms are used. Corticosteroids can also be combined and used concurrently with Mannitol in severe cases.

The products most commonly used by veterinarians are either **dexamethasone** (Azium) or the methylated forms of **prednisone** or

prednisolone (Medrol). These rarely cause any serious side effects as they are only used for a relatively brief period to get the animal through the incident. As soon as the clinical signs pass or at least decrease, treatment is discontinued. It must be remembered that in most of these cases, if the medications fail to achieve their goal, the animal may be paralyzed or lose its life. For a complete discussion of steroids, please refer to chapter 10, and to chapter 11 for non-steroidal anti-inflammatory drugs.

MOTION SICKNESS

Motion sickness is typically associated with excess drooling and, in many cases, vomiting. The dog will be anxious, nervous, and may shake or quiver over the entire body. Some animals may show these signs even before actually being in the vehicle. This, along with other features of the syndrome, leads many veterinarians to believe that motion sickness may actually be a response to fear or apprehension and not motion.

There is therefore no set treatment to control these problems in the dog. Different veterinarians often choose totally different medications. There is no wrong or right answer. The drugs most commonly chosen are either antihistamines or tranquilizers, although others are used.

ANTIHISTAMINES

Orally administered antihistamines are also used in human medicine to control motion sickness as well as other conditions. Two of the most common of these over-the-counter antihistamines are **diphenhydramine** (Benadryl) or **promethazine** (Dramamine). In dogs, it is believed they are effective because they have strong antivomiting (anti-emetic) effects in areas of the brain and inner ear that are responsible for balance and motion detection. These medications are available over-the-counter without a prescription.

In the dog, the dosage varies from animal to animal, with amounts up to 50 mg being given every eight hours. For a more complete discussion of antihistamines and their effects, please see chapter 12.

TRANQUILIZERS

Some veterinarians choose tranquilizers, believing that calming or sedating the animal will be much more effective. It is hoped that the animals will be calm but still able to eat, drink, and walk on their own. The product most frequently prescribed is **acepromazine** (PromAce). This product comes in both an injectable and tablet form, with the latter typically being dispensed to be used on an "as needed" basis when traveling. After being given orally it usually takes an hour or so to take effect and then lasts for six to eight hours. With acepromazine, the owner will notice that the gums and mouth appear dry and the third eyelid more prominent.

There are some unwanted side effects with acepromazine. Because of this, the medication should only be given under the direction of a veterinarian. Epileptics or dogs with other seizure disorders should not be given this medication. It tends to cause a higher frequency of, and potentially more severe, seizures. Additionally, there is a very small percentage of dogs that become more excited and a few may even become vicious. These latter two problems, however, are relatively rare.

Diazepam (Valium)

Valium is utilized by some veterinarians for motion sickness. It has the same general effect as the tranquilizers do, i.e., the calming of the animal without any known true motion sickness effects. An advantage of Valium over the acepromazine-type medications is that it can be used by patients with a history of seizures. Additionally, it is not known to cause hyperexcitability or aggression. However, it is a controlled substance and potentially abusable by humans. Therefore many veterinarians are reluctant to use this product on a routine basis.

SEIZURE DISORDERS

Seizures are a common occurrence in dogs. Obviously only a small percentage of canines have them, but they are far from rare. In most conditions, seizures are related to abnormal activity within the central nervous system, especially the brain. Neural transmissions within the brain go on constantly in a very controlled and coordinated fashion. Anything that disrupts or destabilizes any part of this system may cause a seizure.

The term **epilepsy** is commonly used to describe a disease in which seizures are the most notable feature. An epileptic typically has no abnormal behavior other than the seizures. Unfortunately, epilepsy is not a simple, well-defined disease.

It is actually termed **idiopathic epilepsy,** meaning a seizure disorder of undetermined cause. Presented with a dog suffering from seizures, a veterinarian does every imaginable test from blood work to X rays to CAT scans and can find no detectable physical or physiological abnormality. The diagnosis is then idiopathic epilepsy.

We do have a fairly good understanding of this condition in dogs. Most cases that we work with fall into one of two categories. The first is in certain breeds in which there is a strong genetic pattern for the condition. One generation will pass it on to the next with predictable regularity. These animals will typically have their first seizure before three years of age.

The **grand mal** seizures will initially be very mild, lasting a few seconds to minutes. The animal will become glassy-eyed, lose awareness of the surroundings, and may fall over and paddle with its legs. Over time, the seizures become more frequent and severe. Without treatment, they last for three to ten minutes, with the animal showing all the above signs with more violent thrashing and possibly the loss of fecal and urinary control. There is no set pattern, however, and some dogs might lose control of their bladder, etc., on their first seizure. As any of these dogs continue to mature, in a portion the seizures will continue to worsen, becoming more violent and/or frequent and more difficult to control with medication.

A second, much less common group of epileptics will have seizures that are secondary to or caused by some other unrelated medical condition. They may follow being hit by a car or other possible head trauma. One of the most common causes of seizures in humans is head trauma and, while the relative incidence is different in the dog, it is still a frequently noted aftereffect. It is believed that scar tissue which affects neural transmissions has formed within the central nervous system. In others, the seizures may be related to medical problems within the liver, kidney, heart, or other organ. In some, the seizures may be caused by an abnormality in the formation of the skull.

Medications to control seizures are divided into two categories. There are those used in emergencies and those used for long term maintenance. Emergencies do arise in which the patient is in a prolonged seizure or slips from one to another. These are referred to as **status epilepticus** and are life threatening. The animals may have difficulty breathing, vomit with the potential of inhaling the regurgitated food into their lungs, or simply not come out of the seizure until they finally die of exhaustion or overheating. To bring the seizure under control, drugs are given either intravenously or intramuscularly. If successful, the medication causes the animal to go from a state of perpetual seizure to one of unconsciousness as with an anesthetic. When the animal finally wakes up, the seizure has passed and the animal is normal. Some of these convulsions may not be related to any form of epilepsy but be brought on by poisoning or other medical conditions possibly not related to the nervous system.

On the other hand, long term or maintenance therapy for an epileptic patient, once initiated, goes on throughout the remainder of the animal's life. It is typically an oral tablet or capsule that is administered one to three times per day.

INJECTABLE MEDICATIONS

Phenobarbital and Pentobarbital
For status epilepticus, these are two of the most commonly used products. They are safe and their action is predictable. In most cases, an anesthetic plane is reached within seconds. These are both barbiturate compounds. There are other similar medications in this class that are also used by veterinarians for grand mal seizures.

Diazepam (Valium)
Many practitioners utilize this medication in its injectable form by itself or in conjunction with the above barbiturates. It usually has a longer duration of activity and some feel the animals wake up more smoothly over a longer period of time. To further increase the length of its activity within the body, a portion of the dosage may be given intramuscularly.

Sernyline Derivatives (Ketamine)
This is an anesthetic cleared for use in cats and is one of the most commonly used products in feline medicine. Although not cleared for use in dogs, many veterinarians use this medication to control grand mal seizures in the dog with great success. It is safe, has a rapid onset of action, and with experience becomes quite predictable.

ORAL MAINTENANCE THERAPY TO CONTROL SEIZURES

The goal of anticonvulsant medication use is to eliminate completely or greatly reduce the frequency and severity of seizures. The medications do this through the same mechanisms of action as the products used to control emergency status epilepticus situations. Once dogs go on maintenance products, they generally receive them daily for life. Over time, the dosage may need to be altered. In most cases, the disease gradually increases in severity, therefore requiring higher levels of medication to control the problem. The clinician, working together with the owner, always tries to use the smallest quantity necessary to reach the desired level of control. In many epileptics, even with this type of therapy, we are not able to completely eliminate all seizures all the time. In these cases, we attempt to decrease their frequency and minimize their effect or severity.

After the diagnosis of idiopathic epilepsy has been reached, it would seem obvious that all of these patients would immediately go on some sort of therapy to eliminate the convulsions entirely. Unless the seizures are severe (lasting a long time or in some way being life threatening), this is generally not the case. Rather, we generally wait until they are occurring at least once a month. There are several reasons for this.

Typically, owners bring their animals into a veterinary clinic for examination or treatment when the first seizure occurs. Understandably, these usually frighten the owners much more than they do the dogs. In fact, some veterinarians try to "talk their clients through" the first occurrence over the phone rather than have the patient brought into the clinic. In the vast majority of these cases, during the early stages of this disease the convulsion will pass and the animal will be perfectly normal within a few minutes. Most clinicians prefer to do a physical examination combined with a battery of blood tests as soon as possible following the incident. In the case of the idiopathic epileptic this only eliminates other known seizure-causing disorders, leaving the veterinarian with a diagnosis of exclusion. Remember, there are no tests that can be run that say, "This patient is an epileptic." All that can be said is that the dog had a seizure and in many cases it may never have another one. Therefore, most clinicians prefer to see some pattern or at least a certain frequency before medication is started.

Additionally, there really is no set dosage for the anticonvulsant medications. We have guidelines to use when first putting an animal on these products, but all they are is a starting point. We alter dosages to fit the needs of the dog. To eliminate the seizures, a small dog might take several tablets per day of a particular medication while a much larger dog could be perfectly maintained on a half tablet once a day. Additionally, we cannot even predict with certainty which medication should be used on which dogs. None of the different anticonvulsant medications work equally well on all dogs. In some dogs, one will work fine while another medication may have little or no effect. Also, after time, an animal may become unresponsive to a particular drug and will have to be switched to another one. In every patient, it is a case of trial and error. Therefore, if a patient has had one seizure and there is not another for a year, it is very difficult to determine the correct medication and the appropriate dosage for that animal.

Once the disease has progressed to the point at which the seizures are either life threatening or are occurring at a rate of at least one per month, one of the following medications is chosen to control the problem. Once treatment is initiated, veterinarians would hope to eliminate the seizures completely. In some cases this is not possible and the goal is then to greatly decrease their frequency and severity.

While there are other anticonvulsant products utilized in canine medicine, with some being brought over from the human field, the following comprise over 95 percent of all used today.

Phenobarbital

Today, after years of usage, this is still the preferred anticonvulsant medication in dogs. When compared to other medications used for this purpose, it is by far the least expensive, causes the fewest side effects, is fast acting, has a long-lasting effect within the body, and in most cases does a good job of controlling the seizures. Many owners are not initially concerned about the cost of medications capable of eliminating or reducing the frequency or severity of convulsions in their pets, but when they realize that the animal may be on these products several times a day for life, cost frequently becomes a significant factor.

The tablets are very small and easily given orally. The medication is absorbed by the intestine and works to stabilize activities within the brain, thereby lessening the frequency of seizures. Phenobarbital is metabolized by the liver to an inactive form that exits from the body in the urine. Following initial oral administration, it usually takes a day or two to reach therapeutic levels.

When a patient is initially placed on phenobarbital, the most common side effect is sedation. Some animals will also drink and eat more than normal, urinate excessively, and may seem dizzy or wobbly on their feet. Usually within a week or two, as the body adjusts to the medication and the liver becomes better at breaking it down, these signs are no longer seen. If serious side effects are to be seen with phenobarbital usage, they relate to liver toxicity. These problems are usually eliminated quickly if the animal is taken off this product and switched to an alternative medicine.

Phenobarbital does speed up liver activity and, when used concurrently with other medications that are normally broken down by the liver, this may cause them to be metabolized more rapidly, therefore requiring them to be given at a higher dosage. It does this to certain antibiotics such as chloramphenicol and doxycycline, corticosteroids, antiparasitic drugs such as metronidazole (Flagyl), and certain heart medications such as digitoxin. It is also reported to decrease the absorption by the intestine of the commonly used antifungal product griseofulvin. All in all, this is considered to be a safe and effective product.

Primidone

This is also a very commonly used product, especially on larger dogs. It is, however, not unique when compared to phenobarbital. **Primidone** is usually administered in a tablet form although a liquid is available from human pharmacies. It is absorbed by the intestine, travels to the liver, and is there converted into phenobarbital. Therefore it has the same action as phenobarbital. It is typically utilized at a dosage of 10 to 50 mg/kg per day divided between three doses and given every eight hours. It usually takes several days before effective levels are reached.

Primidone is not as popular as phenobarbital because it is more expensive, has no unique properties over phenobarbital, should be given every eight hours, and its long term usage is recognized to be much more toxic to the liver. Since it is converted to phenobarbital it has the same side effects during the early stages of treatment and the same interactions with other drugs.

However, a percentage of the dogs that suffer from seizures are better controlled with primidone than with phenobarbital. This typically seems to be members of the larger breeds.

Phenytoin (Dilantin)

Just as primidone is often the choice for larger breeds, phenytoin seems to be more frequently used on smaller dogs. It is usually chosen by veterinarians for patients in which phenobarbital or primidone have failed to achieve the expected level of seizure control. This certainly is not a hard and fast rule and some practitioners may recognize certain characteristics in individual cases that cause them to choose phenytoin first.

It can be purchased in tablet, capsule, or liquid form for oral administration. The initial dosage is 10 to 30 mg/kg, with a maximum daily dose of 100 mg/kg. It takes at least a week of administration before therapeutic levels are reached within the body. It is often combined with phenobarbital and used in cases in which the latter medication has failed or no longer controls the seizures adequately. Together, the two augment each other's effects.

Phenytoin is considered much more toxic to the liver than either phenobarbital or primidone. It is rapidly broken down by the liver, causing it to have a short life in the body; therefore it should be given three times a day. It is often poorly or inconsistently absorbed by the intestinal tract, leading to unpredictable amounts making their way into the body. Commonly observed side effects when the animal is first introduced to the medication may include dizziness or uncoordinated gait, increased drinking and urination, vomiting, and shaking over the entire body. Most of these can be eliminated by lowering the dosage. Long term use can cause an overgrowth of the gums. These disadvantages, plus its higher cost, make it less likely to be the product first chosen for use in the epileptic dog.

Diazepam (Valium)

Although **diazepam** is very useful in the control of status epilepticus, it is less satisfactory for long term maintenance. It is effective within a few hours after the first oral dose, but when used in a routine daily fashion, most dogs develop a tolerance to the medication as their bodies get better at breaking down and eliminating it. Most practitioners utilize diazepam orally only when they are first starting a dog on long term anticonvulsant therapy. Many of the other anticonvulsants take several days to weeks to build up therapeutic levels within the body. During this initial period, diazepam will control the seizures until the other product has reached its maximum effect. At that time, diazepam is discontinued.

Diazepam is given as a tablet every twelve hours at a dosage of 0.2 to 0.5 mg/kg. Some patients will show sedation with incoordination, while others may become excited.

Potassium Bromide
Potassium bromide is often used in conjunction with some of the anticonvulsants listed above when their effect is less than satisfactory, or to lower the amount needed to control seizures. It takes prolonged use before the benefits are realized. In most cases, at least two months of continuous therapy are required before an appreciable effect is noticed.

TRANQUILIZERS AND SEDATIVES

Acepromazine
In canine medicine, the medication most typically dispensed by veterinarians for oral use is **acepromazine.** This product also comes in a liquid injectable form, but that is typically restricted to use within a clinic or hospital situation. It is typically used in a tablet form that takes about one hour to take effect and then lasts for six to eight hours when given orally.

Acepromazine belongs to a group of chemicals referred to as the **phenothiazine derivatives.** There are several related tranquilizers used in veterinary medicine also belonging to this group. Others are **chlorpromazine, promazine,** etc. These all work on the brain by slowing the activity of the higher neural centers, producing a calming effect. Acepromazine and these other substances also have some effect on the motor abilities of the animal, making its movements seem awkward or uncoordinated. Owners also often notice that the third eyelid at the inside corner of the eye seems to become more prominent. This is caused by a relaxation of muscles in this area.

In the vast majority of times acepromazine is used, it works exactly as expected. The medication is said to be **hypotensive;** that means it lowers the patient's blood pressure. In most instances, this is of little significance. However, if an animal suffers from a concurrent heart problem or was in shock, this could be dangerous. Additionally, *the product should never be used in those suffering from seizure disorders such as epilepsy.* It lowers the threshold for these periods of abnormal neural activity and potentially causes the patient to have *more seizures* that may also be *more severe* than normally experienced by the patient. *In a small percentage of animals, it may make them more excited and even aggressive instead of calming them.*

Valium

Also known as **diazepam,** this medication is occasionally used in veterinary medicine as a tranquilizer or sedative. Its calming effects are usually not as predictable or consistent as acepromazine but it can be used safely in patients suffering from seizure disorders.

Phenobarbital

This medication is more typically used to control seizures in epileptic patients but can be used as a sedative in dogs and cats. As with Valium, its use is not as predictable as acepromazine, but it is favored in situations in which the patient does suffer from diseases such as epilepsy.

One problem that prevents the more common usage of Valium and phenobarbital is that they are potentially abusable and therefore are controlled substances. This restricts their distribution and causes many veterinarians to be reluctant to use these products.

LOCAL ANESTHETICS

We feel that it is outside the scope of this book to go into most of the anesthetics that are typically used in canine medicine. We will limit our discussion to the local anesthetics that owners may be asked to use on their dogs.

These are applied topically to the skin in an attempt to reduce pain or discomfort. They are found in preparations used to treat hot spots, ear infections, etc. Examples would be **lidocaine, procaine,** or **tetracaine.** Simply stated, they block the ability of the nerve endings that are responsible for detecting pain and touch to be stimulated. These are very safe products and can cause no problems when used as directed.

The Urinary System

The dog's urinary tract is composed of the **kidneys, ureters, bladder, urethra,** associated **blood vessels** and **nerves**, **vagina** in the female, and **prostate** and **penis** in the male. (See Figures 20-1 and 20-2.) Medical disorders affecting these structures are very, very common. Animals of any age can be affected, as can members of any breed. Additionally, in the older dog, kidney failure (synonymous with "renal failure") is a very common cause of death.

Blood is filtered in the kidneys. The waste products of metabolism, certain electrolytes, and some water are collected and excreted through the ureters into the bladder. The bladder is a reservoir where urine is stored before leaving the body. Upon elimination, urine passes through the urethra and exits through the vagina or penis. In the male, the prostate gland surrounds the urethra and is inside of or directly in front of the pelvic bone. This accessory gland produces secretions that are important for sperm viability during breeding.

The most common medical conditions affecting the dog's urinary tract are **bladder infections, bladder stones, incontinence,** and **renal failure.** Each of these can be treated with various forms of medical therapy to eliminate or attempt to control the disorder. In some cases surgery may also be utilized.

BLADDER INFECTIONS

ANTIMICROBIALS

Although a **bladder infection (cystitis)** can be caused by many different kinds or types of microorganisms, most are the result of

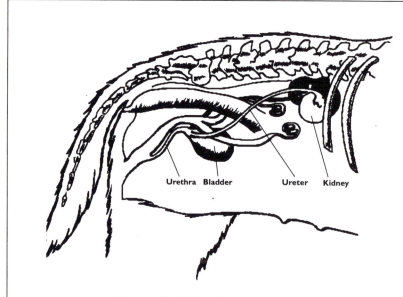

Figure 20-1: Female urinary system.

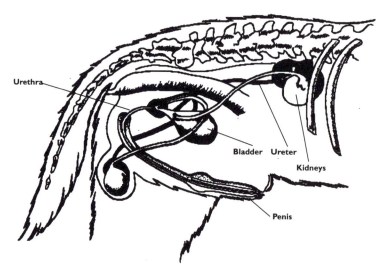

Figure 20-2: Male urinary system.

bacteria which gain access to the bladder through the blood or by migrating up through the urethra. Antimicrobials such as antibiotics or sulfa medications are commonly used to treat these infections.

The same rules apply to the selection of medications as for other areas of the body, with a few exceptions. It is always best to isolate the causative organism through culturing and then do sensitivity testing (see chapter 4) as an aid in choosing an appropriate antimicrobial. However, when treating infections of the bladder, the product must be one that is excreted through the urine unchanged, so that effective levels of therapy are reached *inside* the bladder. Drugs commonly used to treat cystitis would be **amoxicillin, ampicillin, tetracycline, trimethoprim-sulfa,** and the **cephalexins.** Treatments with these usually last from one to three weeks.

URINARY ACIDIFIERS

Cystitis therapy is often directed at affecting the pH of the urine. The majority of all bacteria that cause cystitis do better in an alkaline environment, i.e., with a pH of greater than 7.0. With bladder infections, the urine produced is typically alkaline. Therefore, in a further attempt to control the growth and replication of the bacteria, medications called urinary acidifiers are given orally. They are excreted by the kidneys and **acidify** the urine, i.e., lower its pH to less than 7.0. There are three acidifiers commonly used in canine medicine; they are sold generically or under one of many different brand names. These are **vitamin C (ascorbic acid), d-l-methionine,** and **ammonium chloride.** The dosage required to effectively alter the pH of the urine may vary, and is affected by the severity of the cystitis and/or the diet of the animal.

BLADDER STONES (UROLITHIASIS)

Dogs commonly form stones in their bladders. These can vary in size from that of the head of a pin to larger than a baseball. Stones can also form in the kidneys, but this is very rare in dogs.

Sometimes no outward signs are noted by the owner and a diagnosis is made during a routine physical examination when the veterinarian palpates the animal's abdomen. In many cases, the animal may strain to urinate or urinate frequently passing only small quantities of urine each time, and/or pass blood in urine.

Minerals that pass from the blood through the kidneys leave the urine and bond together, forming stones in the dog's bladder. Stone formation occurs because of metabolic abnormalities that concentrate these minerals or salts in higher than normal levels within the urine. To a lesser degree, stone formation may be more common if the acidity of the urine is such that it causes the minerals to precipitate out more easily.

TREATMENT AND PREVENTION OF BLADDER STONES

Two different scenarios exist with bladder stones. In one case they are present and must be dealt with, while in other animals they have been previously removed and now therapy is prescribed to prevent their reccurrence.

Removal of stones can be done surgically or with the use of special commercially formulated diets (e.g., Hill's S/D or U/D diets) that actually dissolve the stones over time within the dog's bladder. Please refer to chapter 24 for a discussion of prescription diets.

Bacterial infections are common with bladder stones and are controlled through antibiotics. Please refer to the above discussion dealing with bladder infections, or chapter 4, which pertains to antibiotics in general.

Prevention is accomplished by altering the body's metabolism at the kidney level so that the minerals in question are not passed into the urine at such high levels. There are different kinds of stones found in the canine bladder, with different mineral compositions. The most commonly encountered are composed of **struvite, urate, cystine,** or **calcium oxalate.** The particular type often cannot be determined until the stone is removed and tested by a laboratory. The preventative therapy used varies as to the kind of stone formed by the individual dog.

Certain stones form in an alkaline urine (struvite); with these, urinary acidifiers (such as those described above in the section on bladder infections) may be used. Other types of stones such as the calcium, urate, or cystine types are most frequently formed in an acid urine. When attempting to prevent these, medications such as sodium bicarbonate or potassium citrate are used to make the urine more alkaline. These are sold under these generic names or under several different brand names.

Sometimes specialty medications are used to prevent further stone formation. Most of these are also used in human medicine. Examples of these would be:

Allopurinol
This drug is used in dogs that form urate stones. **Allopurinol** (Zyloprim) prevents the formation of the uric acid that is then metabolized to the urates to form these stones.

D-Penicillamine
D-penicillamine (Cuprimine) is used in cases in which cystine stones are formed. It prevents cystine crystalization so that stones cannot form. This product is not well tolerated by some animals, as they may experience gastrointestinal upsets such as vomiting and diarrhea. If this occurs, the product's dosage must be lowered or discontinued.

TREATING URINARY INCONTINENCE IN THE DOG

As dogs age, it is very common for urinary incontinence to develop. Affected animals will involuntarily leak urine. This will be most common while they are resting or asleep, but can happen anytime. The owner may notice that the area where the animal sleeps is damp or smells of urine. These dogs may also lick and attempt to clean the hair and skin around their vaginal and penile openings.

Urinary incontinence in dogs is most common in spayed females, because spaying removes the ovaries and uterus where many of the female hormones are produced. It is believed that these hormones, especially estrogen, help to strengthen the muscle tone of the valvular area at the base of the bladder. A weakness in this area permits small quantities of urine to leak into the urethra and out the vagina.

MEDICATIONS USED TO TREAT INCONTINENCE

Estrogen Supplementation
For years, the only product used to treat incontinence in dogs was **estrogen,** dispensed in a tablet form of the chemical **diethylstilbstrol.** Typically this is sold under a generic label without any brand or trade name associated with it. This medication is much more effective in females than in males. In fact, estrogen eliminates

urinary incontinence in over 98 percent of all affected females. The medication is still widely used today by many veterinarians. However, because of the potential side effects of the estrogenic compounds, other products have gained favor in the last few years.

Estrogens, especially at higher doses, can put an end to new red blood cell production, resulting in a fatal anemia. In unspayed females, they can bring the animal into heat, increase the incidence of a disease of the uterus known as **pyometra,** or stimulate mammary tumor growth.

Testosterone

The male hormone **testosterone** is naturally produced in the testicles of the dog. In some male dogs, whether or not they have been neutered, testosterone is used to successfully treat incontinence. Long-acting injectable products are used. Side effects such as an increased incidence of tumors and hernias have been reported with these preparations. These same tumors and hernias are naturally seen in unneutered males that have not received testosterone treatments.

Phenylpropanolamine

Today this may be the medication most commonly used to treat urinary incontinence in both male and female dogs. It may be dispensed under the trade name Ornade, or the veterinarian may direct the client to purchase some of the over-the-counter human diet medications containing the same active ingredient. Some animals treated with phenylpropanolamine display signs of hyperactivity, but this is uncommon.

MEDICAL MANAGEMENT OF RENAL FAILURE

As long as just one half of one of the body's kidneys functions correctly, an animal or human is fine. But when more than 75 percent of total kidney tissue fails to adequately carry out the tasks assigned to it, the individual slips into renal failure.

The **kidneys** are responsible for eliminating waste products of cellular and protein metabolism from the blood system. Additionally, they help to maintain the body's levels of electrolytes, such as calcium and phosphorus, within narrow ranges. As they fail, **urea,** which is a common by-product of protein metabolism, builds up within the blood system, causing a toxic state we refer to as **uremia.**

The elimination of this compound is one of the main reasons dialysis is used for patients suffering from compromised kidney function. Additionally, the body's electrolyte balances become altered, leading to serious, life threatening conditions as muscles and other structures can no longer function correctly. The acid-base balance of the body is usually affected in these patients and the pH of the body becomes too acid. All or any of these changes typically cause the patient to have gastrointestinal upsets and feel nauseous, which may prevent the individual from consuming adequate food and water.

To help correct these problems, dogs suffering from kidney failure are typically placed on low protein diets, encouraged to consume adequate amounts of food and water, and treated with one or more medications designed to correct the various imbalances within the body. None of these treatments are able to reverse the changes that have occurred within the kidney. They cannot cure the condition. Rather, they are utilized in an attempt to allow the body to function as well as possible with the diseased organs. Once initiated, their use is usually continued for the life of the patient.

MEDICATIONS USED TO REVERSE ELECTROLYTE IMBALANCES

Patients in renal failure are hospitalized and placed on intravenous fluids to flush out their bodies and to correct possible simultaneous dehydration. If they are to return to any form of normal existence at home, electrolyte imbalances must also be returned to normal levels and then maintained with continuous therapy. The two consistent changes seen in renal failure are elevated blood levels of phosphorus and depressed levels of calcium. These changes greatly affect muscle and bone activity and development.

CORRECTING PHOSPHORUS LEVELS

In some patients this can be handled by simply decreasing the amount of phosphorus consumed in the diet. As most cases of renal failure progress, medications are used that prevent phosphorus from being absorbed from the gastrointestinal tract into the bloodstream. These are referred to as **phosphorus binding agents.** They are mixed with or given at feeding times.

These are formulated using either calcium or aluminum. In veterinary medicine either may be used. Some veterinarians prefer the medications containing calcium, as they are inexpensive and help to correct the lower blood calcium levels also common in renal failure. Some are concerned with the use of the aluminum products as they have the potential of leading to forms of aluminum poisoning, but on the other hand, others prefer the aluminum types because they are concerned that the calcium types may lead to dangerously elevated levels of calcium. The calcium-containing products commonly prescribed are generic formulations of **calcium carbonate** or **calcium acetate.** Examples of those containing aluminum would be Amphojel or AlternaGel. Either of these groups can probably be used with little concern if occasional blood work is done to check the quantity needed to effectively lower blood phosphorus levels. The animal must be observed and tested to ensure that calcium or aluminum problems are not developing.

As we stated, blood calcium levels are typically depressed in dogs suffering from kidney failure. Admittedly there are cases in which this is not true, and in some instances, calcium levels may even be higher than normal. Before any calcium therapy is initiated, *it is therefore important that blood tests be done to accurately determine levels within the individual patient.* In those needing supplementation, calcium carbonate or calcium acetate are typically used. These are usually sold as generics listing only the ingredient, not under a trade name.

Correcting the Acid-Base Balance

The body usually becomes too acidic in kidney failure. This causes abnormalities in respiration, gastrointestinal upsets, weakness, and decreased activity levels. Animals suffering from acidosis often feel so poorly that they go off food and water, which further exacerbates their condition. This is usually corrected, *under a veterinarian's direction,* with nothing more than orally administered baking soda, which is **sodium bicarbonate.** As with medications used to correct electrolyte imbalances, its use is constantly monitored to determine the quantity necessary.

Diet Alterations for Patients Suffering from Kidney Failure

There are several factors that must be taken into consideration for the diet of the kidney patient. The most obvious is the overall reduction in the *level of protein* in the diet. Not only must the protein portion of the total diet be reduced, but also the actual size of the protein molecules used. Small protein molecules are much easier for the body to utilize and they produce fewer urea by-products that must be eliminated by the kidney. This decreases the kidney's work load and causes fewer urea compounds to build up in the blood, thereby preventing many of the toxic signs associated with renal failure. Today, excellent commercially prepared diets are available in a wide range of formulations specifically for the kidney patient. See chapter 24 for a discussion of these products.

Please remember that patients suffering from renal failure may, and usually do, have a poor appetite. Human dialysis patients often complain of nausea and have little interest in food. Some of these problems are brought on by the body's acidosis, noted in kidney disease. In the dog, especially in the early stages of treatment, we sometimes use medications to offset these signs in an attempt to increase the quantity of food and water consumed by the patient.

Cimetidine (Tagamet) is often used with these goals in mind as it lowers the acid produced within the stomach, thereby decreasing general body acidosis. Additionally, coating agents such as Pepto-Bismol or Kaopectate can be useful in certain patients. Low dosages of corticosteroids may be used to stimulate the appetite. They have a euphoric affect on some patients, making them feel better and thereby increasing their appetite. In most patients, the effects of the low protein diets, electrolyte-correcting agents, and elimination of acidosis take away the need for many of these additional products.

SUMMARY

All of the urinary tract problems may require long term therapy. Dogs with cystitis often have repeated bouts of the disorder. Stone formations need lifelong treatment and monitoring in most cases. Once renal failure is diagnosed, treatment becomes a priority in the care of the animal.

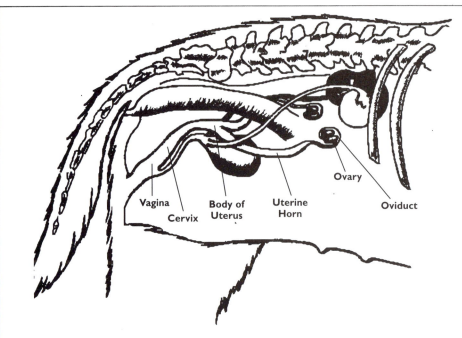

Figure 21-1: Female reproductive system.

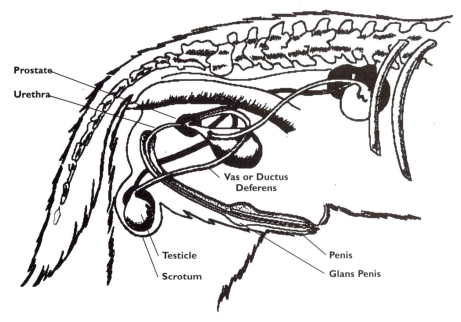

Figure 21-2: Male reproductive system.

CHAPTER 2 1

The Reproductive Systems

The canine male reproductive system is made up of the **testes, epididymis, vas deferens, prostate gland,** and **penis.** In the female it includes the **ovaries, oviducts, uterus, cervix,** and **vagina.** Neutered males lose the testes and epididymis while spayed females lose the ovaries, oviducts, and uterus. The reproductive systems of the intact male and female dog are shown in Figures 21-1 and 21-2.

The reproductive systems of the dog have both unique *and* similar problems when compared with other body systems. Infections are common and are caused by the same organisms that affect other areas. The only difference with the reproductive systems is that to be effective, the antimicrobial medication must be able to reach the infected tissue. In some examples (such as the prostate gland of the male), because of the blood supply and tissue type, it is difficult to get therapeutic levels of these medications into the affected areas. Therefore, specific products must be chosen that are carried into these areas. In the case of the prostate gland, it has been shown that **erythromycin, chloramphenicol,** and **Tribrissen** easily penetrate the gland while most other antimicrobials do not.

Inflammations also occur in the reproductive systems; steroids and nonsteroidal preparations are used when treatment is necessary. Steroids can cause abortions in the pregnant female and must therefore be chosen with care.

Many medications have their action specifically directed at the reproductive systems. In most cases these are only used for intact, unsterilized animals. Their activity is directed at the reproductive process. They may be used to facilitate breeding in males or females that are sterile or suffering from decreased willingness to breed. In other situations, they may be used as contraceptives, preventing females from cycling so they do not come into heat.

CONTRACEPTIVE MEDICATIONS

Dogs can be prevented from breeding by surgical procedures. While tubal ligations are possible, they are usually not preferred by either owners or veterinarians. In the female, the surgery most commonly done is the **ovariohysterectomy,** which removes the ovaries, oviducts, and most of the uterus. This sterilizes the female and prevents any further heat cycles. In the male, a **castration** is done, which removes the testicles and epididymis. Sterilization in the male, when done at an early age, usually prevents them from responding to females in heat.

Today there are medications formulated and approved for contraception in female dogs, but none for males. Those for females can be used when the female comes into heat, or can prevent heat cycles altogether.

Megestrol Acetate

This contraceptive tablet is sold under the brand name Ovaban. It is also sometimes prescribed by veterinarians in the human form, Megace. **Megestrol acetate** is chemically related to the naturally occurring female hormone progesterone. Its activity is related to how it mimics normal progesterone, which means that it often causes an effect opposite to the one caused by estrogen. Ovaban and Megace can be given with or without food, on a full or empty stomach.

In the bitch it is used in several different ways, but there are three common uses. These are **proestrus** treatment, **anestrus** treatment, and to eliminate a **false pregnancy.** The first two prevent breeding while the latter one deals with a reproductive system problem in which breeding did not occur.

In the proestrus treatment, females are placed on Ovaban in the first stage of a heat cycle. This stage is referred to as proestrus. The animal is usually just showing signs of vaginal swelling or bleeding. The medication is then used for eight consecutive days. The female, in most cases, then stops bleeding in three to eight days and does not cycle into the breeding stage referred to as **estrus.** It is still a good idea to prevent them from coming in contact with males as a successful mating is still possible, although very unlikely. The female goes out of heat, not to cycle again for two to nine months.

Anestrus is defined as a period of the heat cycle when the animal's reproductive system is quiescent, i.e., there are no outward or physiological indications of being in heat. In the anestrus treatment, the female is placed on megestrol acetate for thirty-two consecutive days, starting at a time when she is showing no signs of heat. This prevents her from cycling during the thirty-two-day period. Additionally, she may not cycle for another two to nine months, although the majority will come into heat between four and five months after the medication is discontinued.

False pregnancy (**pseudocyesis)** occurs following a normal heat cycle in which the female was not mated or, if breeding did take place, she did not become pregnant. In a false pregnancy, the body responds to abnormal hormonal output and incorrectly takes on many of the behavioral and physical qualities of a pregnant dog. Commonly noted signs in these animals are a swollen abdomen, milk produced by the mammary glands, nesting behavior, carrying toys and other inanimate objects around as if they were newborn puppies, and even encouraging these toys to nurse. This often becomes more than a behavior problem, as infections of the uterus and mammary glands can occur. While most false pregnancies pass uneventfully, others are prolonged affairs.

Megestrol acetate can be used to eliminate a false pregnancy. As soon as this condition appears, the bitch is placed on the medication for eight consecutive days. In most cases, the physical and behavioral signs quickly disappear.

There are certain instances when megestrol acetate should not be used. *It should not be used on a female's first heat cycle.* This can cause problems with reproductive development and subsequent heat cycles. It should not be used in two successive heat cycles or in pregnant dogs.

A final time when this product should not be used needs to be explained further. Breast cancer is very common in the dog. In some breeds it may be the most commonly encountered malignant tumor of the unspayed female dog. Dogs that have breast cancer often see accelerated growth of these tumors following heat cycles. It was therefore assumed that megestrol acetate would be useful in females with these tumors, as it could be used to prevent cycling. However, it has been shown that the medication may also stimulate additional mammary tumor growth in dogs with this disease.

Mibolerone

Mibolerone is sold in a liquid form for oral administration under the brand name Cheque drops. It is approved for long term use in the female dog to suppress estrus or heat activity. It functions by suppressing ovarian activity, thereby eliminating estrus or heat cycling. Chemically, it is considered a nonprogesterone steroid. It is an androgenic compound and therefore closely related to the male hormone testosterone. It can be given with or without food in the liquid form.

Female dogs can be treated for long periods of time with this product, even up to two years. At that time the animal should be removed from the product for several months before therapy is initiated again. When used for long periods of time, the product is expensive and a considerable number of problems have been reported with its usage. Some animals have experienced adverse effects such as liver problems, physical enlargement of the vagina and clitoris, vaginal discharges, body odor, and excess tearing. Behavioral abnormalities have also been noticed, such as sexual mounting of other dogs and aggression. Because of these problems, many veterinarians prefer not to prescribe the product. Additionally, it should not be used on pregnant or nursing dogs, young animals that have not cycled, or animals with a history of liver problems. It should not be used in Bedlington Terriers because this breed has a genetic predisposition to chronic and progressive hepatitis.

MISMATE TREATMENTS

Female dogs frequently breed against the wishes of their owners. It is possible to spay the female at this time, but the problem can be handled medically if the animal is seen by a veterinarian within a few days of the mating. Injections are given to prevent the pregnancy from continuing. An abortion does not occur, but rather the fertilized eggs that pass into the uterus fail to attach to its wall and the eggs die.

The product typically used for this is **estradiol cypionate,** known as **ECP.** A single injection of ECP is given and, in the author's experience, nearly 99 percent of cases of mismatings are terminated uneventfully. The injection does extend the dog's heat cycle, sometimes for an additional two weeks, and she must therefore be contained so a second breeding cannot occur. Additionally, no attempt should be made to breed the female during that heat period.

At the dosages used today problems rarely occur with its use in mismatings. In the past, higher concentrations were used and this could lead to medical problems. Specifically, pyometra would develop, often causing the dog to require a spay (ovariohysterectomy).

MEDICAL TREATMENT OF PYOMETRA

Pyometra is a medical disorder of a female's uterus. This organ has two horns and a body. Uterine horns attach to the ovaries while the uterine body joins the cervix. (See Figure 21-1.)

In the nonpregnant bitch this organ is three to six inches long and about the size of a lead pencil. If pyometra develops, the uterus enlarges to six to ten times this size. It is filled with a combination of white blood cells and fluid discharge from glands lining the wall of the uterus. This material starts to break down, with poisons (toxins) being released into the bloodstream. As these wastes build up in the animal's system, this can lead to death. The contents of the uterus look exactly like the pus that is expelled from an abscess. In most animals this condition progresses, with the uterus enlarging until it finally ruptures. This causes immediate **peritonitis,** an intra-abdominal infection which if untreated leads to the death of the animal.

If caught early in the syndrome, this problem can be handled medically or surgically. An ovariohysterectomy can be done and the problem eliminated. However, in valuable breeding bitches, medical therapy is used in an attempt to save the female's reproductive future. The **prostaglandins** are used, specifically prostaglandin F2alpha. This breaks down the corpus luteum on the ovary which is considered important in initiating and maintaining pyometra. This is only a part of the therapy, as the uterus must usually still be drained surgically. Antibiotics are also administered to these patients, as the uterine contents are often contaminated with bacteria. At this time, prostaglandin F2alpha is not approved for use in dogs, but its use is now fairly widespread.

WHELPING ASSISTANCE

Occasionally bitches in the process of giving birth to their puppies fail to have adequate contractions. They may show little or no effort or have fewer contractions than necessary to expel the pups through the birth canal. In these instances, veterinarians or breeders under the direction of veterinarians, will administer **oxytocin** injections. They can be given intramuscularly, subcutaneously, or intravenously to stimulate and strengthen uterine contractions.

There must be sufficient blood levels of estrogen for oxytocin injections to function correctly. This is not a problem, as there are large estrogen surges from the ovaries before and during labor. The hormone remains in the body for several hours to days after secretion. The major danger with oxytocin is that it may be administered when a puppy is too large or incorrectly positioned for normal birth, and this is mistaken for uterine inertia. In these cases, only a cesarean section can allow birth.

Additionally, many breeders and veterinarians prefer to administer oxytocin injections after the last pup is born to further shrink the overall size of the uterus. This shrinking is thought to help clean the uterus of any remaining placental remnants.

Oxytocin is also used to stimulate and increase milk flow immediately following whelping. Some bitches do not release their milk immediately and injections at this time can be very helpful.

MEDICATIONS USED FOR HEAT STIMULATION AND MODIFICATION

There are many reproductive hormones and chemicals that are used to treat infertility problems or to alter or stimulate heat cycles in the female dog. Some of these same products are used to stimulate sexual activity or interest in both the male and female dog. They are very specialized injectable products and beyond the scope of this book. To be complete, however, some are listed here. They are **luteinizing hormone (LH), follicle stimulating hormone (FSH), pregnant mare serum (PMS), diethylstilbestrol (DES), progesterone, prostaglandins,** etc.

CHAPTER 22

The Endocrine System

The endocrine glands produce **hormones.** These travel in the bloodstream and affect tissues elsewhere in the body.

Hormones are specific in their actions and each hormone exerts its effects on specialized cells that are capable of responding to that hormone. Examples of glands that produce hormones include the **pituitary, thyroid, adrenal, pancreas, ovaries, parathyroid,** and **testicles.** All of these glands produce hormones that exert their effects elsewhere in the body. Although these glands have other important functions, this chapter will only deal with the hormone-producing capacity. Hormones either in excess or in insufficient quantities are harmful and prevent the body from functioning normally. In the canine, the three glands most likely to fail in hormone production are the thyroid, the pancreas, and the adrenal glands. These three glands commonly require medication to help control or supplement their hormonal output.

THYROID GLAND

The **thyroid** gland is a small butterfly-shaped gland located in the throat area. It lies flat against the trachea near the larynx. The principal function of the thyroid gland is to produce the hormone **thyroxine.** It does this by combining the amino acid **tyrosine** with iodine, forming thyroxine.

Thyroxine is normally referred to as **T4.** T4 is basically tyrosine combined with four molecules of iodine. Once T4 is produced by the thyroid and secreted into the bloodstream, it must undergo a

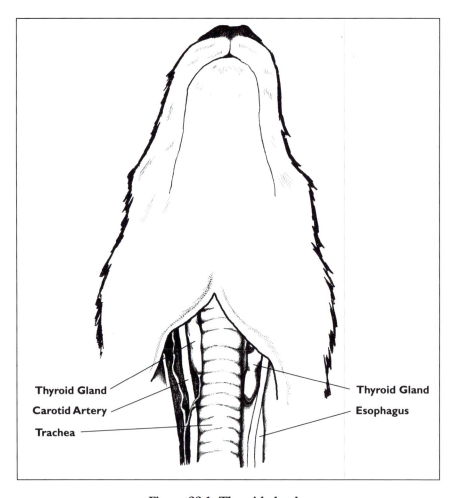

Figure 22-1: Thyroid glands.

chemical process to remove one of the iodine fractions, thus creating **T3,** *the active form of thyroid hormone.* T3 is the form of the hormone that is capable of exerting control over other cells. It is very important in regulating many body functions including the metabolism of nutrients, energy levels, blood pressure, weight control, hair production, fertility, and body temperature.

If the thyroid produces insufficient quantities of T4, or if the body cannot convert T4 to T3 by the deiodinization process, then the body is functionally deficient in thyroid hormone. A **hypothyroid** patient is one that either produces too little thyroxine (T4) or produces adequate quantities but cannot convert it into the chemically active form T3. To treat the hypothyroid patient, it must be determined whether the patient has a production or conversion problem with thyroid hormone. Veterinarians, with the help of specialists called **endocrinologists,** can analyze laboratory blood tests to differentiate a thyroid deficiency due to production from one of faulty conversions. Once a determination and evaluation of hypothyroidism is made, several drugs are available to replace the needed hormone.

L-Thyroxine (Levothyroxine—T4)

The majority of hypothyroid canine patients are treated using a daily dosage of **L-thyroxine.** It is sold under the brand name Synthroid or as the generic form Soloxine. L-thyroxine is T4 as described above and needs to be converted by the body's deiodinization process to the active T3 form. In a patient not capable of the deiodinization process, T4 (L-thyroxine) would not be the replacement drug of choice.

L-thyroxine is administered once or twice daily. In most patients the liver and other cells can store L-thyroxine and release it slowly throughout the day. A once daily supplementation is adequate in these patients. In a few individuals the response is better if the L-thyroxine supplementation is divided into two daily doses. The selection of a once or twice daily administration is based on the individual patient response.

Synthetic L-Triiodothyronine (Cytobin)

L-triiodothyronine (Cytobin) is T3. *It is the active deiodinized form* and therefore does not require the body's capability to deiodinize the T4 molecule. L-triiodothyronine is used in patients that cannot convert T4 to T3. It must be noted here that rarely is T3 used alone. It is given in combination with T4. Some cells such as those of the brain require T4 be converted to T3 within the cells. These nerve cells have a poor ability to absorb orally supplied T3.

With T4 or T3 as a daily supplement, it is possible to overdose the patient, actually causing too much hormone or **hyperthyroidism.** The signs of hyperthyroidism include increased thirst and urination. Additionally, the patient may be hyper or nervous and may even lose weight. Once supplementation begins, follow-up blood tests will help confirm the final amount of supplementation needed. Once the overdosage is corrected the associated signs disappear. Thyroid supplementation is usually for life and periodically the dose may need to be adjusted, usually upward as the thyroid gland continues to fail.

THE ADRENAL GLANDS

There are two adrenal glands, one near each kidney, in the canine. The glands are small, about the size of garden peas. Each gland is made up of two parts, the inner core (**medulla**) and the outer shell, called the **cortex.** The medulla produces two hormones called **adrenaline (epinephrine)** and **noradrenaline (norepinephrine).** These two hormones help to control heart rates and blood pressure, among other things.

The cells of the outer layer or adrenal cortex produce three **steroid hormones. Aldosterone** helps regulate sodium and water loss into the urine. The **hydrocortisone hormones,** of which **cortisol** is the best known, help regulate the metabolism of carbohydrates. The third type of hormones produced by the adrenal cortex are the **sex hormones.** In the male these are androgens, and in the female they are estrogens and progesterones.

Occasionally not enough hormones are produced due to failure of cells within the adrenal cortex or those in the brain which stimulate the adrenal glands. This is termed **hypoadrenocorticism.**

Hypoadrenocorticism causing a low level of hormone production may not drastically affect the overall body hormone levels. Certain hormones produced by the adrenal glands are also produced by other organs. Sex hormones, for example, are also produced by the sex glands, the ovaries and the testicles. Usually, hypoadrenocorticism causes a decreased blood level of aldosterone and hydrocortisone (cortisol). This condition in the canine is referred to as **Addison's disease.**

The opposite of Addison's disease is an adrenal disorder in which excessive quantities of hormones are produced, especially the hormone hydrocortisone (cortisol). This is called **hyperadrenocorticism** and is commonly referred to as **Cushing's disease.**

The two described syndromes, Addison's and Cushing's disease, are actually disorders arising from the outer adrenal layer or cortex. The medulla, or inner core, rarely manifests itself in a clinical disorder in

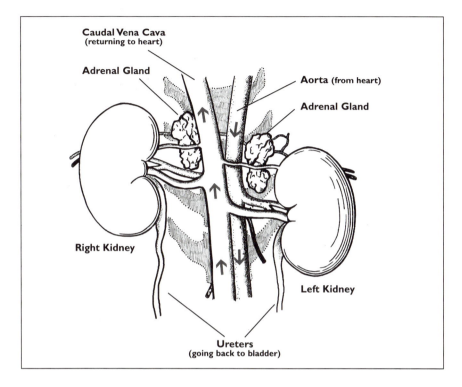

Figure 22-2: Adrenal glands.

the canine. This text will detail the clinical manifestations of Addison's and Cushing's disease and the drugs dispensed to treat them.

ADDISON'S DISEASE (HYPOADRENOCORTICISM)

In Addison's disease, the cells of the adrenal cortex slowly degenerate over time. In many instances this may be the result of autoimmunity, which is destruction of cells by one's own body. The immune system simply recognizes the adrenal cortical cells as "foreign" and therefore attempts to destroy them. Infections of the glands may also destroy the cells and prevent normal functioning. Furthermore, drug toxicities may result in the formation of Addison's disease. Since the hormones aldosterone and cortisol are produced by different cells, there may be varying degrees of clinical manifestation, depending on which cells fail. In other words, the aldosterone-producing cells may fail more than the cortisol-secreting cells and vice versa. In most cases of Addison's disease, both types of cells significantly fail to secrete adequate levels of the hormones aldosterone and hydrocortisone (cortisol). Since this type of Addison's disease is the most common, its therapy will be outlined here. *Addison's disease is best described as low levels of the hormones aldosterone and cortisol.*

Of the three above causes, autoimmunity is the most common in the dog; however, those resulting from drug therapy are the most frequently mentioned.

Steroid drugs such as prednisone and other "hydrocortisone-like" drugs are commonly used to treat or help alleviate many common disorders in the canine, including allergies, arthritis, and other inflammatory ailments. Unfortunately, if these steroids are used at severely high doses they can actually cause the body to suppress the adrenal gland production of normal steroids such as cortisol. When the artificial steroids are removed from therapy, the body fails to stimulate production and is left with a lower than normal adrenal output. This does not provide enough steroids for the body to function normally. It is best if steroids are reduced slowly over time, thus allowing the adrenal glands to respond and restore their normal production levels.

Regardless of cause, the clinical signs associated with Addison's disease are similar. The patient suffering from Addison's disease may have muscle weakness, vomiting, diarrhea, and depression. Because the hormone aldosterone is intimately involved in the regulation of sodium and potassium levels within the bloodstream, these are measured to help confirm the diagnosis. Usually sodium will be abnormally low, with potassium found in excess. Once the diagnosis is confirmed, drug supplementation to replace the low levels of aldosterone and hydrocortisone (cortisol) must begin at once and generally continue throughout life. The most common drugs selected to treat Addison's are fludrocortisone acetate (Florinef Acetate) and prednisone.

Fludrocortisone Acetate (Florinef Acetate)

Fludrocortisone acetate (Florinef Acetate) is a tablet administered daily. It has a dual function in treating Addison's disease in that it replaces the functions of both aldosterone and cortisol. It promotes the retention of sodium and the excretion of potassium to bring them to normal levels. Florinef Acetate may be used as the sole treatment or in combination with prednisone. Administered at excessive levels, it may cause muscle weakness, sodium and fluid retention, and high blood pressure.

Prednisone

Prednisone is a steroid drug used to replace the low level of cortisol. It's available in a wide range of generic forms. In the treatment of Addison's, tablets are administered on a daily basis. Unlike Florinef Acetate, it does not replace the effects of aldosterone. Because of this it is not used alone, but rather in combination with Florinef Acetate. If administered in excess, it can cause fluid retention and excessive thirst, urination, and appetite.

CUSHING'S DISEASE

Cushing's disease results when the adrenal glands are hyperactive and produce excess hydrocortisone hormones, namely cortisol. The overproduction of cortisol may be due to overstimulation of the adrenal glands by the pituitary gland or the hypothalamus within the brain (which stimulates the pituitary gland and causes, in time, hyperactivity of the adrenal glands). The adrenal glands themselves may also cause an excess of hormone production. Regardless of cause, the end result is that the body has an excess of steroid hormones, producing some very characteristic results.

A patient with Cushing's disease generally appears puffy from fluid retention. Additionally, because of the abnormal metabolism of carbohydrates, the body will actually begin burning muscle tissue to get nutrients. This causes a weakening of muscles and, as the abdominal muscles weaken, a pendulous appearance of the abdomen develops. Additionally, the legs may appear thin and weak as muscles atrophy. Thirst and appetite may also be excessive. In severe cases fatty deposits may appear as small whitish clumps within the thin abdominal skin. A generalized hair loss is usually noted over the thorax and abdominal regions.

Drug therapy for Cushing's disease is aimed at actually destroying a portion of the adrenal glands' cells to reduce the output of steroid hormones.

Mitotane (Lysodren)

Mitotane (Lysodren), also referred to as O,P'-DDD, is the most common drug used to medically treat Cushing's disease. Although the exact mechanism of action is unknown, mitotane selectively causes a "dying off" of the adrenal cells that produce the hormone cortisol. The drug is initially administered at a high or loading dose and then is decreased to lower maintenance levels. Mitotane can have side effects, including weakness, vomiting, and loss of appetite.

Ketoconazole

Although normally used as an antifungal agent to treat ringworm and other fungal diseases, ketoconazole is also useful in managing Cushing's disease. It inhibits the production of steroid hormones, including cortisol, estrogen, and testosterone. It has little effect in suppressing the production of the hormone aldosterone. Side effects are minimal, although some patients may experience digestive upsets including vomiting and appetite loss. In some patients, hepatotoxicity is also observed. Ketoconazole is usually selected for use in patients experiencing adverse reactions to mitotane.

THE PANCREAS

The **pancreas** is a small ribbon-like organ that lies along the border of the stomach and small intestine juncture. It has several functions, including the production of digestive enzymes and hormones such as insulin. This particular section will deal with the hormone-producing capacity of the pancreas, specifically **insulin.**

The hormone insulin is necessary to allow the transport of dietary sugar (glucose) into the cells where it can be burned for fuel. Without insulin, glucose simply builds to elevated, toxic levels in the blood. Excessive quantities will be excreted in the urine. The end result is that glucose will not be available to the cells and the patient, in effect, will be starving. Abnormally high levels of sugar (glucose) in the bloodstream can cause unwanted and serious medical conditions such as cataracts and loss of muscle mass and tone.

A failure by the pancreas to produce sufficient quantities of insulin is termed **diabetes mellitus** (sugar diabetes). When the insulin levels are too low (as indicated by high blood sugar and/or urinary sugar), insulin supplementation is necessary. Oral insulin medications used in humans have limited value in the canine and have not

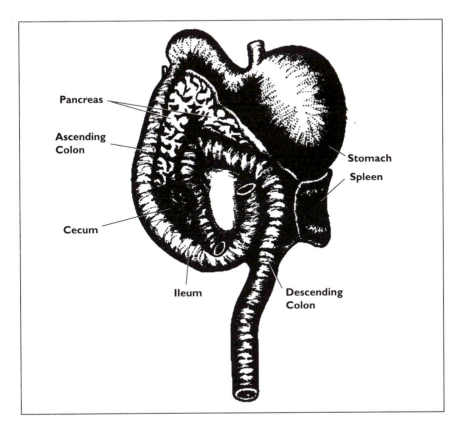

Pancreas

Ascending
Colon

Cecum

Stomach

Spleen

Ileum

Descending
Colon

Figure 22-3: Canine pancreas.

proven a successful treatment. Diabetes is best managed with daily injections of insulin. Insulin is available in several injectable types.

NPH Insulin

Most cases of diabetes in the canine are managed with daily injections of NPH insulin. A single injection of NPH will have its peak effect eight to twelve hours after administration and last up to twenty-four hours. The exact dosage must be determined by a veterinarian. Dosage will vary with diets and activity levels. Different diets contain different levels of sugar. A set feeding regimen and insulin dosage are usually determined prior to releasing the patient from the care of a veterinarian. If too much insulin is administered or not enough food (sugar) is supplied by the diet, then the patient may become **hypoglycemic,** which means the blood sugar is low. The hypoglycemic patient may be weak, delirious, and occasionally suffer seizures. This condition is usually referred to as "insulin shock" or an insulin reaction.

Regular Insulin

Regular insulin has a very quick initial action with a short duration. It is not typically administered at home to manage diabetes in the dog. Rather it is given intravenously during medical emergencies when the blood sugar is severely high. If it is used as a maintenance form of insulin, it is given subcutaneously.

Protamine Zinc Insulin (PZI)

Protamine zinc insulin is a slow-acting insulin of long duration; it may last up to thirty hours. PZI is not commonly used in veterinary medicine as NPH insulin provides a more predictable result.

SUMMARY

Hormone replacement is never simple; the diagnosis for its need and follow-up monitoring are done through blood testing. Owners of animals on these products should understand that retesting will probably be done routinely throughout the animal's life.

PART IV

Nutritional Supplementation

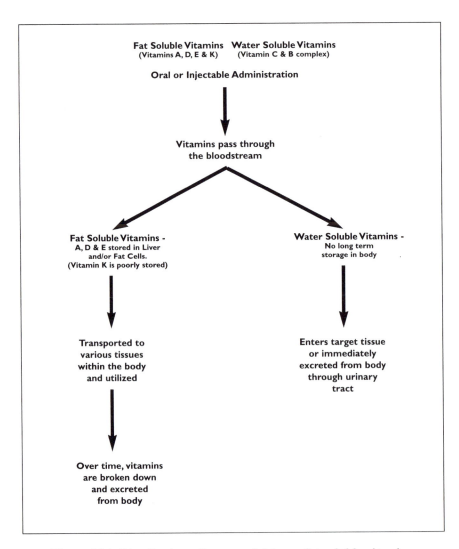

Figure 23-1: Distribution of water soluble vs. fat soluble vitamins.

Vitamins and Fatty Acids— The Essentials of Life

A vitamin is "one of a group of organic substances, present in minute amounts in natural foodstuffs, which are essential to normal metabolism and lack of which in the diet causes deficiency diseases," according to *Stedman's Medical Dictionary*. As defined, vitamins are present in very small quantities in most foods, and it is this fact that leads to the manufacture of vitamin supplements for pets and people. These are very important supplements and, in fact, they are essential for life. The purpose of this chapter is to offer an insight into the major vitamins and what they mean to the normal bodily functions of the canine patient.

The importance of vitamins has been known for only a short time; however, their actual effects were demonstrated centuries ago. The father of medicine, Hippocrates, first advocated using liver to cure night blindness around 400 B.C. We now know that one of the common components of liver is vitamin A and it is the lack of this substance that causes night blindness. Beriberi, the once-feared paralytic disease of humans, was found to be caused by a high quantity of rice in the diet. It is now known that rice is low in the B vitamin thiamine. Low thiamine levels were the real cause of beriberi, and a simple diet change cured the paralysis.

The primary vitamins are normally identified as vitamins A, D, E, K, C, and B complex. Of these A, D, E, and K are the so-called **fat soluble** vitamins, whereas C and the B complex vitamins are **water soluble.** *Fat soluble vitamins are commonly stored in special fat storage cells called* **lipocytes.** *Water soluble vitamins are rarely stored in the body* *except in minute amounts.* Because of this, *fat soluble* vitamins pose the biggest threat if oversupplemented. They are stored in the body, unlike the water soluble ones, which are quickly eliminated via the urine.

FAT SOLUBLE VITAMINS

Vitamin A

The first fat soluble vitamin to be discovered was vitamin A. Vitamin A is known to exist in several forms, such as **retinol, retinaldehyde, retinoic acid,** and the liver storage form **retinol palmitate.** Vitamin A is stored within the liver of the dog. Here it remains until needed by the body. If fed in amounts exceeding the capacity of the liver, it "floats" freely in the bloodstream and excesses can create toxicities.

The main source of vitamin A is the yellow pigment found in plants. This pigment is called **beta carotene.** When fed to dogs, it is easily converted by the intestinal cells into the usable vitamin A.

Not so in cats. Unlike dogs, cats have a greatly reduced ability to convert plant pigment (beta carotene) to vitamin A. Because of this, cats must be fed vitamin A already in the liver storage form of retinol palmitate. This fact is very important in the proper formulation of supplements. Too often pet owners are only concerned with the amounts of vitamin A when in reality the type is most important. For this reason, beware of off-brand vitamin tablets or foodstuffs. Quality is more important than quantity. Enough on this topic for now.

Vitamin A has many roles in the body. It is important for vision and other functions. Deficiencies lead to night blindness, retarded growth, poor quality skin and hair development, and reproductive failure.

To breeders, the vitamin link to growth is of prime importance. The amount of vitamin A needed in the first two years of life is sufficient to warrant supplementation in the diet. Later in life, once full growth is attained, the need for it is still important, but reduced. Lack of vitamin A in puppies and kittens directly relates to low growth rates, muscle weakness, poor vision, and loss of hair coat. In addition, skeletal and nervous disorders such as hydrocephalus and cleft palate are common. Females with inadequate levels of this vitamin will not cycle or ovulate properly and males can become sterile.

It is well established that vitamin A is essential for life. Additionally, a need for supplementation is clear, especially during the growing stages, but vitamin A is one of the two vitamins in which over-supplementation can have negative effects. We have never seen a case of over-supplementation causing toxicosis. In fact, toxicity in dogs has been demonstrated only under experimental conditions. When fed extremely elevated toxic doses of vitamin A, dogs develop muscular weakness and bone abnormalities.

From a practical standpoint, vitamin A supplementation is necessary, especially to the growing puppy or kitten. Infants are born with no liver storage of this vitamin. The first milk (colostrum) is rich in vitamin A and provides an important first source. *Name brand* commercial pet foods are vitamin fortified, and many excellent vitamin supplements are available in tablet, granular, and liquid form. Usually there is no reason to feed more than 12,000 IU per pound of body weight per day.

Vitamin D

Vitamin D is also known as the "sunshine vitamin." Ultraviolet radiation from the sun is important in converting vitamin D into its active D form. This conversion takes place in the outer, most superficial skin layers. Small amounts of vitamin D are also obtained directly through the diet, usually from meat such as liver or fish oils.

A dog's body therefore has two sources of vitamin D: that from the diet and that manufactured in the skin. Vitamin D is an important factor in maintaining proper blood levels of calcium. For this reason, some researchers view it as a hormone rather than a vitamin. For the purposes of this book it will be considered a vitamin. Vitamin D stimulates the kidney conservation of calcium and therefore helps the body to retain it. Because of an interplay with calcium, vitamin D is extremely important in bone formation and nerve and muscle control. Vitamin D deficiencies were very prevalent in the past, but surface only occasionally today. Low levels of vitamin D will cause bone demineralization, as in rickets. Again, supplementation is highly advised both in puppies and, to a lesser extent, in adult dogs. The recommended canine dosage of vitamin D is 11 IU per pound of body weight per day.

Vitamin D toxicities, as with those of vitamin A, are extremely rare. A dog fed excess vitamin D could have abnormal calcium deposits form in the heart muscles and other soft tissues, although this is very rare. Vitamin D plays a major role in skeletal growth, muscle control, and nerve functions. Deficiencies are fairly common and toxicities are rare, if even present.

Vitamin E

Vitamin E is the third fat soluble vitamin. Foods rich in vitamin E include plant oils such as safflower and wheat germ. As with the other fat soluble vitamins, it is highly concentrated in fat and meat such as liver. All vitamin E functions are not known, but it plays a role in the formation of cell membranes and in the metabolism of fats.

Deficiencies of vitamin E will cause cell damage and death in skeletal tissues, heart muscle, testes, liver, and nerves. It is essential in keeping the cells of these organs alive and functioning. Vitamin E deficiencies have been well documented in dogs. The "Brown Bowel Syndrome" is the phrase usually used to describe a dog suffering from inadequate vitamin E. The affected bowels ulcerate, hemorrhage, and degenerate. In addition, the cells of the eye and testes are frequently affected in these animals.

Dog owners commonly read about cats that are fed fish-only diets which are naturally low in vitamin E, causing a syndrome called "Yellow Fat Disease." This does not occur in dogs. Dogs can suffer from deficiencies, but theirs is a different syndrome.

There is no experimental evidence to support the popular belief that vitamin E in excess will help increase stamina in breeding dogs or cats. Vitamin E is occasionally given by owners for this reason, but in the authors' experience, it is not known to be effective.

There are no known vitamin E toxicities in the dog and cat. Fed even at huge levels, no interruption of bodily functions has been demonstrated. Usually 5 IU per day are suggested as the normal cat and dog dosage. This is highly variable depending on the source. The amount is not critical as long as it is adequate. Future research will probably uncover other functions of vitamin E and this may alter the suggested dosage.

Vitamin K

Vitamin K is the last of the fat soluble vitamins. The discovery of vitamin K won the Nobel Prize for Henrik Dam in 1929. From a nutritional standpoint it is important; however, its prime significance in dogs is in the treatment of one of the most common toxicities encountered in animals—rat and mouse poison.

Vitamin K exists in three forms: Vitamin K1 is found in green plants; vitamin K2 is high in fish meal and can be synthesized by the bacteria in the gut; and vitamin K3, also known as **menadione,** is a synthetic precursor of the others. Vitamin K3 is the form most utilized as a supplement. Since vitamin K can be manufactured by the bacteria in the gut of the dog, it is not needed in high levels in food supplements.

Vitamin K is absolutely a must for normal blood function. Without vitamin K, blood cannot clot. Most rat and mouse poisons (a.k.a. Warfarin, D-Con) kill rats and mice by eliminating their ability to clot blood; the rodents internally hemorrhage to death. Contained within the poison is the active ingredient **coumarin.** It is the coumarin that binds to and depletes the body of active vitamin K. Without vitamin K the blood cannot clot and the rodents die. Unfortunately, many dogs and cats accidentally ingest rat and mouse poison and the results are the same. The pet will begin hemorrhaging, usually within the intestinal tract. If the product is chronically ingested in large amounts, then death may follow. If you suspect a pet has ingested this poison, induce vomiting at once and call your veterinarian. If the dog ingests a mouse that has eaten or died because of coumarin, no poisoning will result.

In cases of coumarin poisoning, veterinary treatment will be the administration of vitamin K1, either injected or in tablet form. If instituted early, the patient's life is rarely in danger. Blood transfusions may also be indicated in more advanced cases.

The actual dietary requirements for vitamin K are unclear. The quantity produced by the bacteria of the gut is difficult to determine and this complicates the establishment of supplemental needs. Dietary vitamin K is found in green leafy plants and vegetables.

Vitamin K deficiency in pets has not been documented except in instances of Warfarin toxicosis (rat poison). Likewise, vitamin K toxicity due to oversupplementation has not been reported in dogs.

This concludes the description of the four fat soluble vitamins: vitamins A, D, E, and K. Of the four, only A and D seem to have a potential toxicity and this only experimentally. It is not believed that dogs on today's foods plus typical supplements could possibly have a vitamin toxicosis. The disorders relating to a lack of these vitamins are, however, well demonstrated. These substances are absolutely essential to life. Also understood is the fact that growing animals have much greater requirements than adults. In addition, influences such as lactation, pregnancy, and exercise will all increase the need.

WATER SOLUBLE VITAMINS

Water soluble vitamins are not readily stored by the body tissues, and when fed in excess, they are immediately eliminated from the body via the urine. Because they do not accumulate within the tissues, there is minimal risk of toxic effects. In fact, the authors are not aware of a single toxicity case ever having been documented in dogs. All of the water soluble vitamins, just as with the fat soluble vitamins, are inherently important for life. The lack of adequate amounts has been well described in both pets and people and will be the main focus of the remainder of this chapter.

Vitamin C

Vitamin C has long been considered the "cure" for the common cold in humans. In pets, it has been claimed to prevent hip dysplasia and urinary tract infections and cure feline leukemia.

It is doubted by most researchers that its use will prevent hip dysplasia in a dog that carries the genetic trait. However, most veterinarians have worked with animals that had clinical hip dysplasia who when given high levels of vitamin C, seemed to exhibit fewer signs of joint pain. It does not cure the condition but seems to allow the patient to compensate for or better live with the problem.

In the case of bladder infections, as in human medicine, it is believed that vitamin C is excreted unchanged via the kidneys and therefore acidifies the urine. In most cases, this makes the bladder a much less hospitable place for bacteria to live, as most of the organisms that cause cystitis (i.e., bladder infection) survive much better in environments that have an alkaline pH. Therefore, by acidifying the urine with vitamin C, these organisms are often inhibited or eliminated. This is the reason many people are told by their doctors to drink large quantities of cranberry juice when they have cystitis.

As far as its use in viral diseases like the common cold or feline leukemia, in all honesty, there is little solid evidence of its value. At the same time we would readily admit that vitamin C can do no harm when used. As stated, excesses the body cannot use are excreted unchanged via the urine. Many veterinarians, breeders, and pet owners feel that it helps in the treatment of one condition or another and to these individuals it can only be correct to do what you feel is right.

What we do know is that vitamin C exists in two forms: as **ascorbic acid** and as **dehydroascorbic acid.** Ascorbic acid is easily hydrolyzed (mixed with water) and therefore is readily absorbed through the intestinal wall. Likewise, it easily enters the urine to exit the body. Very little is stored within the body and the minute amount that is stored is contained within the adrenal gland. Ascorbic acid can be fed as a supplement or it can be manufactured within the body from glucose. Unlike dogs, guinea pigs and humans cannot manufacture vitamin C, so their only source is their diet.

Ascorbic acid plays many important functions in bone formation, including bone growth and bone mineralization. Deficiencies of ascorbic acid result in the syndrome known as **scurvy.** Dogs with scurvy exhibit weak bones and swollen joints, usually accompanied by severe tissue hemorrhaging. In young dogs, scurvy is sometimes referred to as **HOD (hypertrophic osteodystrophy).** HOD dogs generally exhibit swollen, painful joints, especially of the limbs. The swollen areas are the portions of the long bones that are actively growing. (It must be added that a lack of vitamin C is only one factor in HOD. There are other causes of HOD that are not related to vitamin C deficiency. A puppy may have HOD, but have perfectly adequate amounts of vitamin C. With this in mind, it is easily explained that only some patients with HOD will respond to vitamin C therapy.)

Vitamin C is definitely justified as a supplement, especially in fast-growing puppies and in lactating bitches. It is not, however, a cure for hip dysplasia. Hip dysplasia is a genetic conformational abnormality and vitamin C cannot alter genetics. It may help alleviate the pain associated with the arthritis caused by hip dysplasia. Whether the dog is in pain or not, or whether vitamin C helps or doesn't, the dog is still dysplastic and should be regarded as such.

Vitamin C has been used with varying degrees of success in helping prevent the formation of some bladder stones in dogs and cats. The vitamin C makes the urine more acidic, which helps discourage the formation of most stone types. Bladder stones are formed as minerals slowly precipitate out of the urine. This reaction is often pH mediated.

In conclusion, vitamin C is widely used as a supplement in growing, pregnant, lactating, stressed, and working pets. There is no concern for toxicity.

Vitamin B Complex

Vitamin B complex consists of a multitude of B vitamins. For purposes of this discussion, **thiamine, niacin, riboflavin, pantothenic acid, pyridoxine, folic acid, B12,** and **biotin** will be detailed. All are B vitamins and together form the water soluble vitamin B complex. Toxicities are not a concern with this vitamin.

Thiamine or **vitamin B1** was the first water soluble vitamin to be identified. It is found in plants, fish, vegetables, fruits, milk, and meats. Like all water soluble vitamins, it is not stored within the body, so it is extremely important that the diet contain a sufficient quantity. Humans suffering low thiamine levels develop a neuromuscular disorder known as **beriberi.** Rice is low in thiamine so beriberi was commonly encountered in rice-eating countries.

In veterinary medicine, a thiamine deficiency is generally associated with pets who are fed a large amount of raw fish. Herring, smelt, and catfish contain large amounts of thiaminase, an enzyme that destroys thiamine. Pets fed these raw meats as their sole source of food will become thiamine deficient. Cooking fish prior to feeding will destroy the thiaminase enzyme and therefore cooked fish poses no problem. A deficiency of thiamine results in weakness and loss of reflexes and nerve control, and eventually causes death.

Niacin, another B vitamin, plays a role mainly in helping enzymes to function properly.

"Black tongue" and "sore mouth disease" are the terms used to describe a dog suffering from a niacin deficiency. Niacin is found in adequate levels in meats and meat by-products and is very low in vegetables and grains. A patient suffering with black tongue will lose weight, fail to eat, and have red inflamed gums, lips, and inner cheeks. Bloody diarrhea and death may follow. Niacin deficiency is generally encountered when owners formulate their own diets for their pets and do not include meat as part of the ration. Be very careful when trying to convert a pet into a vegetarian. Pets are omnivores, which means they must eat meats and "salads." Anything else is incomplete.

Riboflavin is also known as **vitamin B2** and has been proven to be essential to normal growth, muscle development, and hair coat. Riboflavin is found naturally in organ meats and dairy products. It is lowest in grains, vegetables, and fruits. The vegetarian pet is at extreme risk of developing a riboflavin deficiency. Dogs fed a diet deficient in vitamin B2 will have slow or inadequate growth, eye abnormalities, weakness in rear limbs, and eventual heart failure. Deficient patients usually have periodic episodes of fainting; this is termed the "collapsing syndrome of dogs." Riboflavin toxicity from an excess of this vitamin is rare if not nonexistent.

Pantothenic acid is another B vitamin and is found in sufficient quantities in most raw foodstuffs, including meats and vegetables. Processing of foods will reduce the amount of pantothenic acid available to the dog. The role of pantothenic acid has been well described. This acid enables the body to create usable energy from carbohydrates, fats, and proteins. The symptoms of pantothenic acid deficiency include hair loss, diarrhea, and gastric upsets. It has also been associated with early graying, particularly in black-coated animals. There are no known problems with constipation if elevated levels of pantothenic acid are fed.

Pyridoxine is also known as **vitamin B6** and is, therefore, another B complex vitamin. Vitamin B6 is found in many foods but it is easily destroyed by processing. B6 is used by the body in the utilization of amino acids and it is absolutely essential for life. Deficiencies of pyridoxine lead to anemia, poor growth, kidney stones, tooth cavities, skin lesions, and death in advanced cases. There are no known toxicities associated with consuming excess quantities of this vitamin.

Folic acid and **vitamin B12** are two closely related B complex vitamins and are usually discussed together. A deficiency of either can lead to advanced anemia, as they are necessary for production of red blood cells by the bone marrow. White blood cells may also be reduced. Both are usually included in the diet and are found in organ meats. Toxicities caused by the consumption of excessive quantities of these vitamins do not occur.

Biotin is the last of the B complex vitamins detailed here. Biotin is one of the most discussed of all vitamins, primarily because of its role in maintaining healthy skin and hair. It does much more than this, also being necessary for growth, digestion, and muscle function. In some animals, it has been linked to litter size.

Biotin deficiencies have been reported following the consumption of raw eggs. Raw eggs, especially the whites, contain an enzyme called **avidin** that acts to destroy biotin. It is best if raw eggs are not fed to dogs. A patient suffering from a lack of biotin may have poor hair, skin lesions, dried eye discharge, diarrhea, decreased litter size, and in advanced cases paralysis of the limbs. Biotin is found in grains but is not always of a usable quantity. Diets rich in corn or soybeans are best, while those of wheat and barley are deficient. Beef liver supplies the richest source, with brewer's yeast being next highest. Biotin toxicity is rare to nonexistent.

VITAMIN SUMMARY

It should be obvious that vitamin toxicity is extremely rare and there are few known cases. Vitamins A and D show the highest potential for toxicity, but this is not of practical concern. To the contrary, a lack of adequate vitamin intake results in serious health hazards, including death. The pets at highest risk are those that are fed home (or untested) diet formulations. In addition, almost all dogs can benefit from a vitamin supplement and/or a diet fortified with the necessary nutrients. Remember, toxicities are not a problem but deficiencies are. It is suggested that dog owners feed only name brand (tested) supplements and diets unless it is prohibited by specific medical conditions.

FATTY ACID SUPPLEMENTATION

Fatty acids are routinely supplemented in the diets of dogs. This is done to eliminate dryness of the skin and add body, luster, and sheen to the coat, and also for anti-inflammatory and anti-itching relief of any skin disease.

These products are taken orally, absorbed by the body, and carried to the skin by the bloodstream. They are then deposited within the lower or immature layers of the skin and also used by the glandular structure. Their anti-inflammatory properties are believed to be brought about by chemical reactions, converting them to prostaglandins and other substances that have strong anti-inflammatory effects.

How fatty acid supplements actually reduce itching in various allergenic disorders is not very well understood. Their properties have been evaluated by several research studies. The products do eliminate skin dryness and this itself eliminates some itching.

However, while some dogs suffering from allergies favorably respond to these products, a portion show no improvement of the skin. In fact, some even have concurrent oily seborrhea that prevents any dryness.

There are two fatty acids that are routinely used for supplementation, **linoleic** and **linolenic.** They cannot be synthesized by the dog's body and must be included in the diet. They are available in several forms and also in related compounds, such as the other common metabolics within the omega 3 and omega 6 fatty acid groups.

These fatty acids are found in over-the-counter preparations such as Vitacoat, Linatone, Derm Caps, and Vitacaps. There are several other products on the market today. Many animals will respond to one product but not another. The owner of a dog must often try more than one product to achieve the desired effect.

Response is not immediate and any effect will usually be noticed in three to five weeks. These products are naturally deposited in the lower, immature layers of the skin.

The supplementation of these products is done even when a good quality dog food is utilized. There are no known toxicities reported with these products, even at excessively high levels. However, some animals may develop loose stools, especially when the supplement is first given. This is not permanent and will be alleviated by decreasing the amount of fatty acid supplement. Almost all patients can benefit from fatty acid supplementation, at least during certain periods of the year and/or stages in life.

Common Uses and Contraindications of
Canine and Feline Prescription Diets

	Conditions Warranting Use	When Not to Use
k/d diet	Kidney disease Heart disease Liver disease	Breeding females Growing puppies and kittens
u/d diet	Kidney failure Animals that have or may form bladder or kidney stones/crystals consisting of urates, oxalates, cystines, etc.	Breeding females Growing puppies and kittens Animals that have or may form bladder or kidney stones/crystals consisting of struvite
s/d diet	Animals that have or may form bladder or kidney stones/crystals consisting of struvite	Breeding females Growing puppies and kittens Do not use with urine acidifiers Do not use over 6 months without veterinarian supervision Heart disease Kidney failure Do not feed with table scraps or other commercially prepared diets Animals that have nonstruvite bladder or kidney stones or crystals such as those consisting of urates, oxalates, cystines, etc.
c/d diet	Animals that have or may form bladder or kidney stones/crystals consisting of struvite Feline Urologic Syndrome *(i.e. lower urinary tract disease)* Gastrointestinal conditions	Breeding females Growing puppies and kittens Animals that have nonstruvite bladder or kidney stones or crystals such as those consisting of urates, oxalates, cystines, etc. Do not feed with table scraps or other commercially prepared diets
h/d diet	Heart disease Conditions resulting in high blood sodium levels *(esp. those that cause fluid retention)*	Animals suffering from abnormally low blood sodium levels Breeding females Growing puppies and kittens While suffering from vomiting/diarrhea Do not use with urine acidifiers
i/d diet	Gastrointestinal upsets Allergies Liver disease Pancreatic disease	- -
w/d diet	Colon diseases Gastrointestinal upsets Diabetes Prevent weight gain after dieting	Breeding females Growing puppies and kittens
r/d diet	Obesity in mature dogs and cats	Breeding females Growing puppies and kittens Stressed or rehabilitating animals Do not use with urinary acidifiers
d/d diet	Allergic dermatitis Gastrointestinal upset	Breeding females Growing puppies and kittens Do not use with urinary acidifiers
a/d diet	For hospital use only	- -

CHAPTER 24

Prescription Diets—
The Reasons for Those Used

Special manufactured diets can be a part of or the sole component of the treatment of a disease.

You have undoubtedly heard these products mentioned under such designations as **i/d, k/d, u/d,** etc. In most cases, a specific organ system of the body is diseased or failing and having difficulty carrying out normal functions. Its job can be made easier by these special foods. In other situations, the diet may alter the body's physiology and thus prevent it from causing further damage to this organ or system. Although there are several companies producing excellent quality "prescription" diets, in their clinics the authors have utilized those made by Hills. Because of familiarity with this particular line of premade diets, these products will be used as examples for this discussion. Those produced by other manufacturers are similar and have similar usage and results.

Just as people with high blood pressure are advised to stay on low salt diets and diabetics try to limit their intake of candies and other sweets, dogs with certain medical conditions can improve their health or prevent further deterioration by "watching what they eat." That's not easy for them to do. Their preference in foods has been formed through millions of years of development and evolution. They know what they want or prefer to eat but, unfortunately, this may not be what is best for them. Considering some of the disorders that we will discuss, it isn't always easy for us to prepare just what they need in our own kitchens.

KIDNEY DIETS

The first example is renal (kidney) failure, a very common disorder in older dogs. It seems that modern veterinary medicine has made it possible for many of our canine friends to outlive their kidneys. Renal failure in the dog does not mean that the animal cannot produce urine. In fact, the opposite is true. In the early stages of this condition, affected dogs actually produce larger quantities of urine than normal dogs. This implies that the kidneys are no longer able to filter from the blood the various potentially toxic wastes and by-products which have been produced by the body. In any animal, they are excreted in the urine. The kidney failure patient is producing urine but there are not enough wastes being carried out with it.

Renal failure is usually seen in dogs eight years of age or older. These patients have a specific difficulty in eliminating the by-products of protein metabolism. When protein molecules of the dog's diet are digested (broken down into smaller molecules), urea compounds are produced that contain nitrogen. They are very toxic and this is where the term "uremic poisoning" comes from. The kidneys normally remove urea compounds from the blood and expel them though the urine. As the kidneys age and undergo degenerative changes, they lose the ability to complete this simple function. The urea-containing compounds build up to high toxic levels within the blood and other tissues of the body. The amount of toxins in the blood can be measured by laboratory tests such as the **BUN (blood urea nitrogen).**

Some owners incorrectly believe that kidney failure is caused by high protein diets. This is not true. The change that occurs in the kidneys is from natural aging, and/or bacteria and toxins which damage the anatomical structures responsible for removing the urea compounds. Then they simply cannot perform their normal functions. Proteins in the diet do not initiate the problem. However, once the problem is present, they can make it much worse!

Short of dialysis or kidney transplants, there is little we can do for this problem except increase the intake of fluids and alter the diet. The specific prescription diet used in the early stages of kidney failure is **k/d,** "kidney diet." Animals must have some protein in their diets. Most commercial foods use the relatively inexpensive large proteins for this requirement. By using even higher than necessary levels of proteins, the manufacturers provide an additional source of calories or energy at the same time. This less expensive route is fine for most animals but not for the patient with renal failure. The larger the protein molecule, the more times it must be broken down to reach a size that is usable by the body. Each of these steps involves the fracturing of a chemical bond and production of the toxic urea-containing compounds. Smaller proteins require less energy for the body to digest, and also produce much less urea because fewer chemical bonds within the molecule need to be broken. The k/d formula uses very small proteins at the lowest level necessary to fulfill the needs of the body. This significantly decreases the kidneys' work load because there are lower levels of the urea compounds within the blood. To compensate for the loss of calories, the carbohydrate and fat levels within the k/d are increased. This diet also has reduced levels of sodium and phosphorus, which further decreases the work load on the kidneys and the rest of the body.

k/d is used by veterinarians in the treatment of liver diseases as well, because this organ is one of the main sites of protein metabolism and breakdown. By decreasing the total quantity of protein in the diet and utilizing higher quality proteins that are easier for the system to work with, the liver is also spared. Additionally, k/d may be used in cases of heart failure. In these situations, the kidneys often do not receive the normal quantities of blood because the blood-pumping abilities of the heart are decreased. Therefore, the kidneys have less blood available to filter in their attempt to cleanse it of urea compounds. To keep the levels of toxins within the blood at a minimum, k/d may be used. The low sodium (salt) levels also help in preventing high blood pressure, which is hard for a failing heart to deal with.

When a dog in the early stages of kidney failure is placed on k/d, the side effects of this disease are often completely eliminated. The BUN returns to normal levels and the toxicities and effects of uremic poisoning are eliminated. It is important to stress that these diets are an all or nothing option in most cases. Owners cannot add tidbits of steak or other proteins to the diet and expect to get any benefit from k/d. This product is a complete and balanced diet. For it to work optimally, the dog really cannot eat anything else.

If the kidneys continue to degenerate and k/d is no longer able to maintain the blood urea nitrogen at normal or nontoxic levels, the animal is switched to **u/d,** uremic diet. This food has even lower levels of proteins than k/d. It is also very useful in animals with severe liver disease or failure and animals that produce certain kinds of bladder stones. The combination of very low protein and decreased mineral levels aids in the elimination of stone formation. U/d is also a complete diet, and dogs can thrive on it for years if their kidneys continue to function. To get the most benefit, it is very important that the patient be fed nothing else but u/d.

BLADDER STONES

One of the more recent additions to the Hills line was **s/d,** stone diet. As we've discussed before, one of the most common kinds of bladder stones of dogs are those made of struvite. S/d is low in magnesium, phosphorus, and ammonia-producing compounds, all of which are the ingredients of struvite bladder stones. This diet can not only be used to prevent the formation of stones in the urinary tract, but it can also be used to dissolve stones that are already present! This is very important in some cases, as it may eliminate the need for surgery. S/d is a complete diet but only for the short term. Because the mineral levels are very low, it could lead to health problems if used over long periods of time. In our practice we try to restrict its use to periods of no longer than six to nine months. This is an excellent and useful product but, just as the others, you can't expect it to work if you're adding much else to the diet. Also, of the four major kinds of bladder stones, it can only be used successfully in cases involving those made of struvite.

As part of a "one-two" punch against struvite bladder stones, Hills developed Canine **c/d** (not to be confused with Feline c/d), which is designed to prevent stones from forming. It is a complete and balanced diet and can be used as the sole food for years. Not only does it have moderately low levels of the above items that are important for struvite formation, but c/d consistently causes the urine to be acid (instead of alkaline). For struvite to form, the urine must generally be alkaline. Veterinarians therefore use s/d for six months or so to dissolve the stones present, or utilize it following surgery to clean up any small particles remaining, then switch over to Canine c/d as a lifelong preventative. These two diets have significantly decreased the problems and incidence of the most common kinds of bladder stones.

HEART DIET

Canine patients with heart disease basically have the same routines as their human counterparts—diets with low sodium (salt) levels, medications to strengthen the heart, diuretic tablets (which are often referred to as "water pills"), and restricted activity. Hills makes an excellent prescription diet called **h/d** (heart diet) that is low in sodium, therefore helping to relieve problems with water retention and elevated blood pressures. Additionally, since the kidneys of these animals often start to fail or at least are not receiving enough blood for them to do their job correctly, h/d has lower than normal levels of protein.

GASTROINTESTINAL DISORDERS

For intestinal upsets, be they short or long term, Hills has formulated **i/d** (intestinal diet). This is probably one of the most frequently used of all the prescription diets. When dogs suffer from gastrointestinal tract upsets, the last thing we want to happen is for them to ingest anything that excites or irritates the digestive system. (If you had an upset stomach, you probably wouldn't eat a large pizza.) i/d is made primarily of egg, poultry, rice, and corn and is one of the blandest, least greasy dog foods on the market today. It is a complete diet and can therefore be used by itself for the life of the animal. Examples of use would be during or following any diarrheal disease, after intestinal surgery, or while recovering from surgery or long term illness. Additionally, i/d is used with any of the pancreatic diseases. Remember that the pancreas is the organ that produces insulin and the digestive enzymes which function within the intestines. Diets that irritate or inflame the gut will do the same to the pancreas and therefore will worsen any medical conditions affecting this organ. Certain forms of hepatitis are exacerbated with high fat food; i/d is also the preferred diet for animals suffering from these conditions.

Veterinarians attempt to manage diarrhea with i/d, but for constipation we use **w/d,** a high fiber diet. Many incorrectly believe that the role of fiber in constipation is to increase the bulk of the stools and make it easier for the body to pass them. This idea omits one of the primary functions of the large intestine: water balance of the body. Food is prepared for digestion in the stomach, broken down more completely and absorbed in the small intestine, and finally prepared for excretion from the body by the large intestine. At times when the body needs to conserve fluids or prevent excessive loss, the walls of the large intestine absorb more water from the food as it passes through this organ, producing a drier, harder stool. Fiber which cannot be absorbed by the dog draws moisture and tends to reverse this process, increasing the amount of water that remains in the large intestine. The stools are therefore softer and more easily expelled by the body. In the dry form, w/d is between 16 and 17 percent fiber, while a food like i/d is 1 percent or less.

High fiber diets like w/d are also preferred by many veterinarians as a long term management tool for diabetic dogs. Glucose (sugar) from the diet is absorbed through the walls of the gastrointestinal tract directly into the bloodstream. In fact, the body works hard to do this as rapidly as possible, and it can cause wide fluctuations in blood glucose levels. The body naturally regulates these levels with insulin, which moves the sugar molecules from the blood vessels into the body's tissues. The body senses whenever blood glucose concentrations rise, and causes the pancreas to release insulin. Diabetic animals, however, have lower than normal production and we must therefore add insulin to their systems via injections. The artificial additions of this hormone are only done once or twice a day versus the constant release of a normally functioning pancreas. High fiber diets slow the rate at which glucose is absorbed via the intestines into the body, which has a regulating effect. It prevents wide swings in blood glucose levels and produces a more consistent level of sugar in the blood. This makes maintaining a diabetic patient on predetermined levels of insulin much easier. In our practice we have been surprised by the great difference this single dietary step has made on the overall management of our diabetic patients.

w/d is a complete and balanced diet and can therefore be used as a sole ration, lifelong if needed. Because of this, veterinarians frequently utilize it for weight control in dogs that tend to become overweight. When used for this purpose, it is recommended that the animal first be brought down to what is believed to be the correct weight and then maintained on w/d. It's like losing weight and then putting yourself on a high fiber, bulky diet. You can eat more and feel full.

REDUCING DIETS

Hills produces a food just for dieting called **r/d** (reducing diet). It's high in fiber and low in calories. A cup of dry r/d contains only about 200 calories, while the same quantity of i/d would have about 330, w/d about 220. Compare these to a high fat commercial brand of dog food found on the grocery store shelf at 500 to 650 calories per cup! As with most of the prescription foods, it is available in either dry or canned formulations. This sometimes becomes important since most overweight dogs have been fed a lot of table scraps or canned foods and will accept the canned r/d better than the dry form. When trying to accomplish weight loss in the four-legged best friend, the veterinarian often treats both parties. When an owner is sent home with something that the pet will not eat, the animal simply waits, knowing that the owner has been trained to recognize the fact that the dog is not eating and needs something special. As expected, the owner will frequently step in and liven up the r/d with something to encourage consumption. The added gravy, ice cream, or whatever defeats the purpose of the reducing diet. So, by starting out with the more readily accepted canned r/d and later switching to the less expensive dry form, success may be achieved in reducing Fido. If it works, the veterinarian would then switch to w/d to help keep the weight off.

Diet and weight loss are really no different in dogs than in people. While you and I might go to the grocery store and purchase a cart full of 200 calorie microwave meals and then starve ourselves, it would be better to simply increase our time spent exercising and decrease the time spent eating. r/d and w/d are good tools but they are not the only answer. As many as 90 percent of the dogs that cross the door of our clinic don't get the exercise they need!

ALLERGY PROBLEMS

For dogs with food allergies, **d/d** has been developed. It was one of the first lamb and rice products on the market and is a very good quality diet that helps in the management of many food allergies. However, we shouldn't confuse food allergies with the much more common ones brought on by inhaled pollen grains, flea bites, synthetic or natural rug fibers, straw, house dust, etc. Nor will this food solve a food allergy if the patient is allergic to lamb, rice, or anything else found in the d/d formulation. In some dogs it's the answer, but for others it does no good at all.

INTENSIVE CARE NEEDS

One of the newest of the prescription diets is **a/d,** but it is usually restricted to use in a clinic situation. It's a liquid preparation that can be tube fed and is most commonly used for recovering or convalescing patients. a/d is a highly concentrated source of calories, is easily digested, and is especially worthwhile in those cases where dogs will not or cannot eat on their own.

SUMMARY

That completes the discussion of the prescription diets currently available. They are very effective if used in the right situation, but that also means the owner must be willing to feed *only* the canned or dry preparation *as it is.* Remember, if anything is added to increase the desire of the pet to eat, it will usually defeat the purpose of the formulation. By the way, owners don't need a prescription to buy many of these foods, and they are beginning to show up on the shelf at pet stores. Still, it is recommended that you talk to your veterinarian before using any of them.

Glossary of Terms

Abscess—a small pocket-like collection of white blood cells, usually forming as a result of a localized infection.

Aerosol—a liquid solution dispensed as a mist by compressed air.

Allergen—a substance, such as pollen, which is capable of inciting an allergic response or hypersensitivity.

Anabolic—the process in which energy is used to make chemical compounds from smaller units.

Anemia—a lower than normal number of red blood cells in the bloodstream.

Antibiotic—a substance produced by one microorganism that can kill or inhibit the growth of another. Usually used to help destroy bacteria.

Antibiotic resistance—the resistance of a microorganism to antibiotics.

Antibody—a protein produced by the tissues to fight foreign substances that enter the body, such as bacteria and viruses.

Antifungal—an agent that destroys or inhibits the growth of a fungus.

Antihistamine—a drug that counteracts the effects of histamine; usually used to combat the effects of allergies and motion sickness.

Anti-inflammatory—an agent that combats inflammation.

Antimicrobial—an agent that kills or inhibits the growth of a microorganism.

Antitussive—an agent that causes a decrease in the severity and/or frequency of coughing.

Aqueous humor—the fluid found within the eyeball which provides nourishment to the interior eye structures and keeps the eyeball inflated.

Arrhythmia—a variation from normal heart rhythm.

Arthritis—an inflammation of a joint or its surfaces.

Ataxia—a lack of muscle coordination, usually causing an abnormal or staggered gait.

Autoimmune disease—a disease in which one's own body produces antibodies against its cells, and the body destroys its own cells.

Bactericidal—an agent that kills or destroys bacteria.

Bacteriostatic—an agent that inhibits the growth of bacteria.

Beta blockers—a group of drugs that block the effects of adrenaline. Usually this slows the heart rate and constricts the arterioles supplying the skeletal muscles. Commonly used in patients suffering from cardiac abnormalities.

Bradycardia—an abnormal slowing of the heart rate.

Catabolic—a process taking place in which a chemical is broken down into smaller units, producing energy.

Chemotherapeutic—a therapy utilizing drugs or chemicals to protect the body.

Colitis—an infection or inflammation of the colon.

Colostrum—the antibody-rich first milk produced immediately before and after giving birth.

Coma—being in a state of unconsciousness.

Contraception—the prevention of pregnancy, usually with hormone therapy.

Debilitated—a condition of weakness and poor overall health.

Dermatophyte—a fungus living upon the skin. Although not a worm, members of this group are generally referred to as causing ringworm.

Diuretic—a substance used to increase urine production.

Ectoparasite—a parasite that lives on the outside surface or skin of another animal. Ectoparasites include fleas, ticks, lice, and mange mites.

Eczema—an inflammation of the outermost layers of skin, usually creating itchiness, redness, and flaking.

Electrolyte—a chemical substance capable of conducting an electrical current. Examples include sodium, potassium, calcium, and chloride.

Endocrinologist—an authority on glands and hormones and their actions on the body.

Fatty acids—a combination of hydrogen, carbon, oxygen, and glycerol. Fatty acids play a principal role in hair and skin health.

Fogger—a canister used to dispense an insecticide in a fog-like mist. Often associated with treatment of houses for fleas.

Fungicide—a drug that kills fungi.

Fungistatic—a compound that slows or impedes the growth of fungus.

Generic drug—a drug sold not under a brand name, but often only named for the active ingredient.

Giardia—a protozoan that parasitizes the intestines of animals, often resulting in diarrhea.

Gluconeogenesis—a process in which the body, especially the liver, manufactures the sugar glucose from non-sugar sources such as amino acids and fats.

Gram negative—a term used to describe bacteria that resist permanent staining in the laboratory. The staining properties help identify bacteria types.

Gram positive—a group of bacteria that absorb a chemical stain in the laboratory. The retention of certain stains helps to identify bacteria types.

Hepatitis—an inflammation or infection of the liver.

Hepatotoxic—an action destructive to liver cells.

Hip dysplasia—a condition resulting from a misshapen ball and socket joint of the hip.

Histamine—a chemical substance produced by the body to protect it and promote healing. It can also affect blood pressure, heart rate, and stomach secretions, among other things.

Hormone—a chemical substance produced by cells in one part of the body, but having its action on cells in another area of the body.

Hypersensitivity—a term used to describe a greater than normal reaction to a foreign agent such as pollens, flea saliva, etc.

Hypertension—an abnormally high blood pressure.

Hypotension—a decrease in blood pressure.

Infestation—a term used to describe an invasion of parasites.

Insecticidal—a compound that kills insects.

Intracellular—an action taking place within a cell.

Intramuscularly—a term used to describe the administration of an agent directly into the muscle.

Intravenously—a route of administration of a substance into the vein.

Keratitis sicca—an inflammation of the cornea as a result of inadequate tear production.

Mange—an infestation of mange mites.

Mast cell—a cell within the blood that produces chemicals such as histamine and plays a role in allergic responses.

Mastitis—an infection or inflammation of the mammary glands.

Miticide—a preparation used to kill mites such as ear mites and mange mites.

Nephrotoxic—destructive to kidney cells.

Ototoxic—destructive to the structures of the ear.

Pannus—an increased vascularization and pigmentation of the cornea of the eye. Most common in the German Shepherd Dog breed.

Parasite—an organism that lives on or in the tissues of another organism while causing damage to that animal.

Parenterally—a term used to describe the administration of a drug by means other than by mouth.

Pediculosis—an infestation of lice.

Phlegm—a mucous substance produced by the respiratory tract.

Platelets—a group of cells within the bloodstream that function in the clotting of blood.

Pyometra—an infection of the uterus.

Remission—a period of time in which the symptoms of a disease decrease in severity.

Residual—a long-lasting effect.

Ringworm—a term used to describe the circular skin lesions resulting from certain fungal infections.

Seborrhea—an abnormally high production of oils or sebum by the skin glands.

Seizure—a convulsion, often associated with epilepsy.

Sex hormones—hormonal secretions involved in sexual functions. In the male this is testosterone. The female sex hormones are estrogens and progesterones.

Subcutaneously—the administration of a substance immediately under the skin.

Synergistic—a term used to describe the actions of one or more drugs used together giving an effect greater than either drug alone.

Tachycardia—an abnormally high heart rate.

Tranquilizer—a compound that calms a patient.

Urea—the by-product of protein metabolism and degradation. Urea is excreted in the urine, as high levels become toxic to the body.

Urinary incontinence—a phrase used to describe the inability to control urination.

Vasodilators—a group of drugs used to dilate blood vessels to aid in increasing blood flow and/or decreasing blood pressure.

A P P E N D I X I

Drug Dosages

The common dosages for the medications discussed in this book are listed below. They are usually the recommended dosages as listed by the manufacturer or in pharmacological texts. These dosages often vary because of the severity of the condition, interaction with other medications currently being used, or the condition of the patient. Always follow the specific recommendation of your veterinarian. Many topical products such as flea and tick preparations are not listed as they are not "dosed" in that manner.

Medications are usually listed in the metric system, i.e., milligrams (mg) and kilograms (kg). The weight of the dog is listed in kilograms. To convert the weight from pounds to kilograms, simply ~~multiply~~ *divide* your dog's weight in pounds by 2.2 to determine the kilogram weight. Therefore a ten-pound dog would weigh ~~twenty-two~~ *4.54* kilograms (e.g., 10 pounds ÷ 2.2 = ~~22~~ *4.54* kilograms).

The following abbreviations are used:

PO—*per os,* or to give orally
SQ—subcutaneously
IC—intracardiac
IM—intramuscularly
IV—intravenously
ml—milliliter
mcg—microgram
gm—gram
mg—milligram
kg—kilogram (usually the weight of the dog)
mEq—milliequivalents

U—units
IU—international units
rd—recommended dose
bid—twice daily
tid—three times daily
qid—four times daily
q—every, **h**—hour, and **wk**—week. Therefore the listing of "10mg/kg q 12h PO" would mean to administer 10 milligrams per each kilogram of body weight of the patient every twelve hours orally.

acepromazine: 0.56–2.25 mg/kg PO q 6–8h
acetaminophen: 15 mg/kg q 8h PO
acetazolamide: 5–10 mg/kg q 8–12h PO; *glaucoma,* 4–8 mg/kg q 8–12h PO
acetylsalicylate: 10–25 mg/kg q 12h
allopurinol: 10 mg/kg q 8h, then reduce to 10mg/kg q 24h
aluminum hydroxide: 10–30 mg/kg PO q 8h (with meals)
aluminum-magnesium combination: 0.2–0.4 ml/kg PO q 8h
amikacin: 5–10 mg/kg IM IV SC bid or tid
aminopentamide: 0.01–0.03 mg/kg q 8–12h PO
aminophylline: 10 mg/kg q 8h PO
ammonium chloride: 100 mg/kg q 12h PO
amoxicillin: 10–20 mg/kg q 8–12h PO
amphotericin B: 0.25–0.5 mg/kg IV slow infusion q 48h, to a cumulative dose of 4–8 mg/kg
ampicillin: 20–40 mg/kg q 8h PO
ascorbic acid (vitamin C): 100–500 mg/day
atropine: 0.02–0.04 mg/kg q 6–8h, IV IM SC; *organophosphate and carbamate toxicosis,* 0.2–0.5 mg/kg as needed
betamethasone: 0.1–0.2 mg/kg q 12–24h PO
bismuth: 0.25–2.00 ml/kg PO tid or qid
bismuth subcarbonate: 0.3–3.0 gm q 4h PO
butorphanol: 0.55–1.1 mg/kg q 6–12h PO
calcium carbonate: 5–10 ml q 4–6h PO
carbenicillin: 10 mg/kg q 8h PO
cefaclor: 4–20 mg/kg PO tid
cefadroxil: 22 mg/kg q 12h PO
cefixime: 10 mg/kg q 12h PO
cephalexin: 10–30 mg/kg q 6–12h PO
chloramphenicol: 40–50 mg/kg q 6–8h PO

chlorothiazide: 20–40 mg/kg q 12h PO

chlorpheniramine: 4–8mg/dog q 12h PO; maximum rd 0.5 mg/kg q 12h

chlorpromazine: 0.25–0.5 mg/kg q 6–8h PO

chlortetracycline: 25 mg/kg q 6–8h PO

cimetidine: 10 mg/kg q 6–8h PO; *renal failure,* 2–5 mg/kg q 12h PO

ciprofloxacin: 5–15 mg/kg q 12h PO

clindamycin: 11mg/kg q 12h PO or 22mg/kg q 24h PO

cloxacillin: 20–40 mg/kg q 8h PO

cyclosporine: 10mg/kg q 12h PO q 24h; *topical treatment for kerato-conjunctivitis sicca,* 1–2% solution in oil: instill 1 drop in eye q 12h

dexamethasone: 0.25–1.25 mg/kg q 24h PO or 2–4 mg/kg IV

dextromethorphan: 0.5–2 mg/kg q 6–8h PO

dichlorophen: 267 mg/kg PO; repeat in 2–4 wk

dichlorphenamide: 3–5 mg/kg q 8–12h PO

dichlorvos: 26.4–33mg/kg PO

diethylcarbamazine: 6.6 mg/kg q 24 PO

diethylstilbestrol: 0.1–1.0 mg/dog q 24h PO initially and then once weekly

digitoxin: 0.02–0.03 mg/kg q 8h PO

digoxin: 0.005–0.01 mg/kg q 12h PO for maintainance

dihydrostreptomycin: 11–15 mg/kg q 8–12h IM SC

dimenhydrinate: 4–8 mg/kg q 8h PO

diphenhydramine: 25–50 mg/dog q 8h PO

diphenoxylate: 0.1–0.2 mg/kg q 8–12h PO

dipyrone: 28 mg/kg q 8h IV IM SC

d-l-methionine (methionine): 150–300 mg/kg/day PO

doxycycline: 2.5–5 mg/kg q 12h PO

d-penicillamine: 10–15 mg/kg q 12h PO

enalapril: 0.5 mg/kg q 12–24h PO

enrofloxacin: 2.5–5mg/kg q 12h PO or 5 mg/kg q 24h PO

epinephrine: 20 mcg/kg or 0.1–1.5 ml of 1:1000 (1mg/ml) solution or 1–5 ml of 1:10,000 (0.1mg/ml) solution, IV IM SC IC

epsiprantel: 5.5 mg/kg PO

erythromycin: 10–20 mg/kg q 8–12h PO

fenbendazole: 50 mg/kg/day for 3 days PO

fluconazole: 2.5–5 mg/kg q 12h PO

flucytosine: 25–50 mg/kg q 6–8h PO (maximum dose: 100 mg/kg q 12h PO)

fludrocortisone: 0.2–0.8 mg(0.02 mg/kg) q 24h PO

flunixin: 1.1 mg/kg/day 3 day/wk PO

folic acid: 0.004–0.01 mg/kg/day (4–10 mg/kg/day)

furosemide: 2–4 mg/kg q 8–12h or as needed PO; adjust to lowest possible dose needed

gentamicin: 2–4 mg/kg q 6–8h IV IM SC

griseofulvin: 50 mg/kg daily (may be given in divided doses) PO; maximum dose 110–132 mg/kg/day PO in divided treatments

hetacillin: 20–40 mg/kg q 8h PO

hydralazine: 0.5 mg/kg (initial dose) titrated to 0.5–2 mg/kg q 12h PO

hydrocodone: 0.22 mg/kg q 4–8h PO

hydrogen peroxide: *to induce vomiting,* 5–10 ml PO; may repeat once within 10 minutes

hydroxyzine: 2 mg/kg q 4–8h PO

ibuprofen: 10 mg/kg PO q 24–48 h

insulin: *starting dose,* 1 U/kg q 24h SC (titrate to effect)

isopropamide: 0.1–0.2 mg/kg q 12h PO

itraconazole: 2.5 mg/kg q 12h to 5 mg/kg q 24h PO

ivermectin: *heartworm preventative,* 6 mcg/kg q 30d PO; *microfilaricide,* 50 mcg/kg PO 3–4 wk after adulticide therapy; *ectoparasitic therapy,* 200–300 mcg/kg PO—do not use in Collie or Collie crosses; *respiratory parasites,* 200–400 mcg/kg weekly PO—do not use in Collie or Collie crosses

kanamycin: 10 mg/kg q 6–8h IV IM SC

kaolin plus pectin: 1–2 ml/kg q 2–6h PO

ketoconazole: 10–30 mg/kg/day in divided treatments PO; *hyperadrenocorticism,* 15 mg/kg q 12h PO

lincomycin: 15–25 mg/kg q 12h PO

l-thyroxine: 22 mcg/kg PO bid or 0.2–0.4 mg/kg daily in divided doses

l-triiodothyronine: 4–6 mcg/kg PO tid

magnesium citrate: 2–4 ml/kg PO; **hydroxide** (milk of magnesia) *antacid,* 5–10 ml/total dose per day; *cathartic* 15–50 ml PO

mannitol: *diuretic,* 1 gm/kg of 5–25% solution IV to maintain urine flow; *glaucoma or CNS edema,* 0.25–2 gm/kg of 15–25% solution over 15–60 min IV (repeat in 4–6 hours if necessary)

mebendazole: 22 mg/kg (with food) q 24h for 3 days

meclofenamic acid: 1 mg/kg/day PO for 5 days

methscopolamine bromide: 0.3–1.0 mg/kg q 8h PO

methylprednisolone: 1 mg/kg q 1–3 weeks SC IM

metoclopramide: 0.2–0.5 mg/kg q 6–8h PO

metronidazole: 25–65 mg/kg q 24h PO, 12–15 mg/kg q 12h; *giardiasis,* 10 mg/kg q 8h PO; *antibacterial*

milbemycin oxime: 0.5 mg/kg q 30d PO

mineral oil: 10–50 ml q 12h PO

mitotane: *PDH,* 50 mg/kg/day PO (may be given in divided doses) for 5–10 days, then 50–70 mg/kg/wk PO; *adrenal tumor,* 50–75 mg/kg/day for 10 days PO, then 75–100 mg/kg/wk PO (adjust dose based on cortisol measurement)

nandrolone: 1.0–1.5 mg/kg/wk IM

neomycin: 10–20mg/kg q 6–12h PO

nph insulin: typical starting dose 1 U/kg q 24h SC (titrate to effect)

ormetroprim plus sulfadimethoxine: 55 mg/kg on first day and 27.5 mg/kg/day thereafter PO

oxytetracycline: 7.5–10 mg/kg q 12h IV; 20 mg/kg q 12h PO

penicillin G: sodium 20,000–40,000 U/kg q 6–8h IV IM; **procaine** 20,000–40,000 U/kg q 12–25h IM; **potassium** 20,000–40,000 U/kg q 6–8h IV IM

phenobarbital: 2–8 mg/kg q 12h PO

phenylbutazone: 15–22 mg/kg q 8–12h PO (maximum dose: 800 mg)

phenylpropanolamine: 1.5–2 mg/kg q 12h PO

phenytoin: *antiepileptic,* 20–35 mg/kg q 8h PO; *antiarrhythmic,* 30mg/kg q 8h PO

piperazine: 44–66 mg/kg PO once

potassium bromide: 30–40 mg/kg q 24h PO (adjust dose via monitoring)

potassium citrate: 50–75 mg/kg q 12h PO

praziquantel: < 6.8kg body weight: 7.5mg/kg once; > 6.8 kg body weight: 5mg/kg once

prednisolone: 0.5–1 mg/kg q 12–24h PO initially, then taper to q 48h given in AM

prednisone: 0.5–1 mg/kg q 12–24 PO initially, then taper to q 48h given in AM

primidone: initial dose is 8–10mg/kg q 8–12h and then is adjusted to 10–15 mg/kg q 8–12h

procainamide: 20–50 mg/kg q 6h PO (maximum dose: 40 mg/kg)

prochlorperazine: 0.1–0.5 mg/kg q 6–8h IM SC

promazine: 1–2 mg/kg q 6–8h PO

promethazine: 0.2–0.4 mg/kg q 6–8h PO (maximum dose: 1mg/kg)

propranolol: 0.2–1 mg/kg PO q 8h

psyllium hydrophilic mucilloid: 1 tsp/5–10 kg (added to each meal)

pyrantel pamoate: 5 mg/kg PO once, then repeat in 7–14 days

quinidine: 6–20 mg/kg q 6–8h PO

ranitidine: 2 mg/kg q 8h PO

salicylic acid: *analgesic, antipyretic,* 10–20 mg/kg PO q 8h; *anti-inflammatory,* 20–40 mg/kg PO q 12h

sodium bicarbonate: *acidosis,* 0.5–1 mEq/kg IV or as guided by blood gas analysis; *renal failure,* 10 mg/kg q 8–12h PO (adjust as necessary); *alkalinization,* 50 mg/kg 8–12h PO (1 tsp is approximately 2 gm)

spironolactone: 1–2 mg/kg q 12h PO

stanozolol: 1–4 mg q 12h PO; 25–50 mg/wk IM

streptomycin: 20 mg/kg q 6h PO

sulfadiazine: 100 mg/kg PO loading dose, followed by 50 mg/kg q 12h PO

sulfadimethoxine: 55 mg/kg PO loading dose, followed by 27.5 mg/kg q 12h

sulfamerazine: 50 mg/kg q 24h PO for 5 days

sulfamethazine: 100 mg/kg PO loading dose, followed by 50 mg/kg q 12h PO

sulfanilamide: 30–60 mg/kg q 24h PO for 5 days

sulfasalazine: 10–30 mg/kg q 8–12h PO

terfenadine: 4.5–10 mg/kg q 12h PO

testosterone: 1–2 mg/kg q 2–4 wk IM

thiabendazole: 50 mg/kg q 24h for 3 days, repeat in 1 month

thiamine: 10–100 mg/day PO

tobramycin: 2 mg/kg q 8h IV IM SC

toluene: 267 mg/kg PO, repeat in 2–4 weeks

triamcinolone: 0.5–1 mg/kg q 12–24h PO, taper dose to 0.5–1 mg/kg q 48h PO

trimeprazine: 0.5 mg/kg q 12h PO

trimethoprim: 15 mg/kg q 12h PO or 30 mg/kg q 12–24h PO

tylosin: 7–15 mg/kg q 8h PO; *colitis,* 40–80mg/kg/day (with food)

vitamin A: 625–800 IU/kg q 24h PO

vitamin B complex: 0.5–2 ml q 24h IV IM SC

vitamin C: 100–500 mg/day

vitamin D: 500–2000 U/kg/day PO

vitamin E: 100–400 IU q 12h PO; *immune mediated skin disease,* 400–600 IU q 12h PO

vitamin K: *short-acting rodenticides,* 1 mg/kg/day PO for 14 days; *long-acting rodenticides,* 3–5 mg/kg/day PO for 3–4 weeks

Drug Interactions and Contraindications

The usage of drugs and medications in dogs can often cause problems. Sometimes this depends on a pre-existing medical condition in the animal or because of other medications that are being used simultaneously.

Liver and kidney disease are pre-existing medical conditions that most frequently cause problems with the use of certain drugs. Many medications are metabolized or excreted by these organs. If they have been damaged by disease, age, or other drugs, medications that would normally be easily eliminated by the body build up to levels that can potentially cause toxic side effects on the patient they were given to protect.

Examples of other common medical conditions that may predispose animals to develop problems when treated with specific medications are epilepsy, hypothyroidism, heartworm disease, glaucoma, etc.

Most medications can be used simultaneously without causing problems. In fact, often they improve each other's ability to help the patient. There are, however, medications that should not be used together. They may either negate each other's effects or injure the patient because of some interaction.

The following medications, all discussed in this book, can cause potential problems. This should not be considered a complete list of contraindications or interactions, but is limited to the more common or potentially serious ones encountered in canine medicine.

The following letters or abbreviations are used: **(C)** is used for "contraindications," **(I)** for adverse "interactions" with other medications.

acepromazine (C) do not use in dogs with seizure disorders, e.g., epilepsy

acetazolamide (C) do not use in dogs with severe liver or renal function impairment; do not use in dogs suffering from Addison's disease, diabetes mellitus, or that are allergic to sulfonamides

acetazolamide (I) may decrease absorption of primidone by intestine; if used together with primidone or phenytoin, abnormalities of bone tissue may occur; when used together with steroids or diuretics, blood potassium levels may be depressed

acetylsalicylate (C) do not use in animals with a history of gastric ulceration

allopurinol (C) possible problems can occur in dogs with impaired renal function

allopurinol (I) can increase chances of toxicities occurring with the anticancer drug cyclophosphamide; urinary acidifiers should not be used concurrently as they may increase chances of urate stone formation

aminoglycoside antibiotics (C) should not be used in animals with impaired kidney function

aminoglycoside antibiotics (I) concurrent use of diuretics such as furosemide increases the potential for renal toxicity or ototoxicity with the aminoglycosides; do not use concurrently with chloramphenicol, as their actions are antagonistic

aminopentamide (C) do not use in patients with glaucoma or certain forms of heart disease

aminophylline (C) animals suffering from heart, kidney, or liver disease should be monitored carefully while on this medication

aminophylline (I) propranolol's mechanism of action works antagonistically against aminophylline; directly concurrent use of phenobarbital lessens the action of aminophylline; concurrent use of antacids decreases absorption of aminophylline by intestines

amitraz (C) do not use in pregnant animals

ammonium chloride (C) do not use in pregnant animals; preferably not used in animals with severe liver or renal function impairment

amphotericin B (C) extreme care should be taken when used in animals with any impairment of renal function

amphotericin B (I) care should be taken not to use simultaneously with any other potentially nephrotoxic compounds

antihistamines (C) usually avoid use during pregnancy

antihistamines (I) concurrent use with phenothiazine sedatives or barbiturates may have an additive sedative effect on patient; if used simultaneously with phenytoin, activity and potential adverse reactions of phenytoin are increased

atropine (C) animals with concurrent heart problems should be monitored closely when atropine is used (especially when given orally or by injection); do not use in dogs with glaucoma

atropine (I) interactions with numerous medications are noted with atropine but most of these occur with oral or injectable usage and are much less common when used as a solution topically— some increase its activity while others decrease it; during use, the veterinarian should be aware of medications that the patient is on and pre-existing medical problems

butorphanol (C) do not use in pregnant animals or those with a history of liver disease

butorphanol (I) animals should be monitored closely when butorphanol is used simultaneously with phenothiazine tranquilizers or barbiturate anticonvulsants, as sedative effects can be additive

calcium carbonate (C) care should be taken in animals suffering from renal function impairment

calcium carbonate (I) most calcium products decrease the intestinal absorption of phenytoin and the tetracyclines

carbamates (C) do not use in pregnant dogs

carbamates (I) care must be taken when simultaneously using several different carbamates or organophosphates on the dog or its environment, as these are all acetylcholinesterase inhibitors and their additive effect can easily cause toxicities; when phenothiazine tranquilizers are used simultaneously with carbamates they increase the potential for carbamate toxicity

cephalosporin antibiotics (C) patients with impaired renal function should be monitored closely when treated with cephalosporins

cephalosporin antibiotics (I) any medications that also have the potential to harm the kidneys should not be used concurrently with the cephalosporins unless absolutely necessary, as their toxic effects can be additive; chloramphenicol is antagonistic in action to the cephalosporin antibiotics and should not be used simultaneously with them

cholinesterase inhibitors (I) care should be taken when using different preparations containing cholinesterase inhibitors simultaneously, as their potential for adverse side effects is additive; do not use with phenothiazine tranquilizers

chloramphenicol (C) do not use in pregnant dogs or ones with impaired liver function

chloramphenicol (I) inhibits liver metabolism and therefore any other medications that are normally broken down by the liver have their activity increased, as they are not removed from the body (e.g., most of the anticonvulsant drugs); do not use with any members of the aminoglycoside, penicillin, or cephalosporin groups of antibiotics as its action is antagonistic to them

chlorothiazide (I) concurrent use with glucocorticoids may increase the potential for depression of blood calcium levels; in lowering blood calcium levels, chlorothiazide may increase the chances of toxicity problems from digitalis usage

chlorpromazine (C) should not be used in dogs suffering from seizure disorders or tetanus

cimetidine (C) should not be used in dogs with severe impairment of kidney, liver, or heart function

cimetidine (I) inhibits liver metabolism and therefore most drugs that are normally broken down by the liver have their activity increased or prolonged; orally administered antacids decrease absorption and activity of cimetidine

ciprofloxacin (C) do not use in pregnant or lactating dogs; do not use in young dogs or ones with impaired renal function

ciprofloxacin (I) concurrent use of antacids hinders absorption of ciprofloxacin through intestines

clindamycin (C) dogs with impaired renal or liver function should be monitored closely during usage

clindamycin (I) do not use with chloramphenicol as their actions are antagonistic

cyclophosphamide (I) if barbiturates are used concurrently, cyclophosphamide is broken down faster by the liver; cyclophosphamide decreases activity of digoxin if they are used concurrently

cyclosporine (C) dogs with a history of liver or kidney disease should be monitored closely when cyclosporine is taken internally

cyclosporine (I) concurrent use with other nephrotoxic drugs may increase the potential for similar adverse reactions with cyclosporine usage; simultaneous use of drugs that stimulate liver metabolism (e.g., anticonvulsants such as primidone, phenytoin, or phenobarbital) will speed breakdown of cyclosporine by the body when it is taken internally

cythioate (C) do not use in greyhounds; do not use in pregnant animals

cythioate (I) care should be taken when this product is used with other cholinesterase inhibitors as their potentials for adverse side effects are additive

dextromethorphan (I) concurrent use with antihistamines, tranquilizers or other medications that have a sedative effect will increase the drowsiness noted with this product

diazepam (I) if used with other central nervous system depressants, their effect can be additive to that caused by diazepam

dichlorphenamide (C) should not be used in dogs with severe impairment of liver function

dichlorphenamide (I) can potentially interact with and suppress the activity of insulin given to diabetics; prevents normal absorption of primidone by the gastrointestinal tract; concurrent usage with primidone and phenytoin can lead to bone diseases

diethylcarbamazine (C) should not be given to dogs with heartworm disease; should not be used in dogs with impaired liver function

diethylstilbestrol (C) should not be given to pregnant dogs

digitoxin (I) diuretics such as furosemide and the heart medications verapamil and quinidine increase the potential for adverse digitoxin side effects; digitoxin is normally metabolized and broken down by the liver, and medications (e.g., the antibiotics chloramphenicol and tetracycline or the heart medication quinidine) that slow down liver metabolism increase the quantity within the dog and therefore increase the possibility of digitoxin toxicity

digoxin (I) same as those noted for digitoxin

diphenoxylate (I) drowsiness will be increased if used with phenothiazine tranquilizers or barbiturates or other central nervous system depressants

dopamine (I) phenytoin inhibits the action of dopamine

enalapril (C) should not be used in dogs with severe kidney impairment

enrofloxacin (C) do not use in pregnant dogs or in young dogs during active growth periods because of potential damage to developing cartilage and bone

epinephrine (I) antihistamines may increase the effect of epinephrine on the body; it should not be used concurrently with most heart medications

erythromycin (I) do not use simultaneously with penicillins, lincomycin, clindamycin, or chloramphenicol as their antibacterial activities are antagonistic; do not use with terfenadine

fluconazole (C) animals with a history of impaired liver function should be monitored closely while on this product

fluconazole (I) fluconazole increases the activity of phenytoin and may cause dosages to be altered

flucytosine (C) do not use in pregnant animals

flucytosine (I) amphotericin B slows kidney excretion of flucytosine and may therefore increase chances of toxicity problems

flunixin (C) do not use in patients with a history of impaired kidney function or gastrointestinal ulceration

furosemide (C) do not use in dogs suffering from severe renal disease

furosemide (I) risk of increase in potential toxicity side effects from aminoglycoside antibiotics if used concurrently with furosemide; furosemide increases the rate at which many medications are excreted by the kidneys and may cause an increase in the dosage of these products; if furosemide is allowed to depress blood levels of potassium excessively, there is an increased chance of toxicity from concurrently used digoxin or digitoxin

glucocorticoids (C) do not use in pregnant dogs; care should be taken when administered to animals suffering from serious bacterial or viral infections, diabetes, kidney failure, or serious heart disease

glucocorticoids (I) dogs should not be vaccinated while being treated with glucocorticoids; diabetics will probably need higher insulin dosages while on glucocorticoids

griseofulvin (C) do not use in pregnant dogs; dogs with a history of impaired liver function should be monitored closely during usage

griseofulvin (I) phenobarbital inhibits absorption by the gastrointestinal tract

hydralazine (I) concurrent use of this product and propranolol may lead to excessively low blood pressure, causing extreme weakness or fainting; concurrent use with phenylpropanolamine may lead to excessively rapid heart rates

hydrocodone (I) excessive sedation may be noted if used concurrently with other medications that also have the potential to depress, such as phenobarbital, phenothiazine tranquilizers, or antihistamines

ibuprofen (C) do not use in dogs with a history of gastrointestinal ulceration

insulin (I) the following medications used concurrently will decrease the efficiency or activity of insulin or be antagonistic to insulin's actions and may lead to an elevation of blood sugar: glucocorticoids, furosemide, female hormones such as progesterone or estrogen, l-thyroxine; the following medications have the opposite effect and may lead to a decrease in blood sugar levels: phenylbutazone, stanozolol, tetracycline, and propranolol

isopropamide (I) the activity of isopropamide may be increased if used concurrently with phenothiazides, antihistamines, and some heart medications; glucocorticoids and primidone increase the possibility of unwanted side effects from isopropamide

ivermectin (C) should not be used in dogs already infected with heartworm disease; at higher doses than those stated on the label, it should not be used in Collies or Collie crosses

ketoconazole (C) do not use in pregnant dogs; dogs with a history of liver disease should be monitored while this medication is used

ketoconazole (I) all antacids including the antihistamine types decrease the absorption of this product; do not use with terfenadine; phenytoin decreases the activity of ketoconazole

lincomycin (I) the actions of chloramphenicol and erythromycin are antagonistic with lincomycin; the absorption by the gastrointestinal tract of lincomycin is inhibited by coating agents such as Pepto-Bismol or Kaopectate

l-thyroxine (levothyroxine) (C) dogs with severe heart disease should be carefully monitored when placed on l-thyroxine

l-thyroxine (levothyroxine) (I) l-thyroxine increases the metabolic level of most areas of the body and therefore its usage usually causes a need for an increase in insulin dosage

liothyronine (l-triiodothyronine) (C) same as l-thyroxine

liothyronine (l-triiodothyronine) (I) same as l-thyroxine

mannitol (C) extreme care should be taken when administering to dogs with severe heart or kidney disease

mebendazole (C) do not use in dogs with history of liver disease

meclofenamic acid (C) do not use in pregnant dogs or those with a history of gastrointestinal ulceration; do not use in dogs with a history of impaired liver or kidney function

meclofenamic acid (I) should not be used concurrently with aspirin or related medications

megestrol (C) do not use during or before a dog's first heat cycle; do not use in pregnant dogs or those with breast tumors

metoclopramide (C) do not use in dogs with seizure disorders

metoclopramide (I) do not use with phenothiazine tranquilizers; medication inhibits the absorption of digoxin by the gastrointestinal tract

metronidazole (C) do not use in pregnant dogs or those with a history of liver disease

metronidazole (I) the anticonvulsants phenobarbital and phenytoin cause more rapid breakdown of metronidazole and therefore require a higher dosage

mibolerone (C) do not use in pregnant dogs or those with kidney or liver disease; do not use in Bedlington Terriers; do not use before first heat cycle; care should be taken if used in animals with seizure disorders

milbemycin oxime (C) do not use in dogs that are currently infected with heartworm

mitotane (I) mitotane accelerates the breakdown within the liver of phenobarbital and may cause the dosage of this anticonvulsant to be increased; can have a sedative effect on the central nervous system and if used concurrently with other medications having similar action (such as antihistamines, tranquilizers, or barbiturates) their effects may be additive

organophosphates (C) do not use in pregnant bitches; extreme care should be used when administered to sighthounds such as the Greyhound

organophosphates (I) do not use with phenothiazine tranquilizers; care should be taken when using different cholinesterase inhibitors simultaneously, as their potentials for toxic side effects are additive

pancrezyme (I) concurrent use of antacids decreases effectiveness

penicillin antibiotics (I) concurrent use of antacids decreases absorption by the gastrointestinal tract; should not use concurrently with tetracyclines, erythromycin, or chloramphenicol as their bacterial action is antagonistic to the penicillins

phenobarbital (C) care should be taken when used in dogs with history of liver disease

phenobarbital (I) this medication decreases the effectiveness of concurrently used glucocorticoids, quinidine, metronidazole, and chloramphenicol; its sedative or depressant action on the central nervous system is increased if used with phenothiazine tranquilizers or antihistamines

phenylbutazone (C) care should be taken when used in animals with gastrointestinal ulceration; do not use in Scottish Terriers

phenylbutazone (I) do not use with most other nonsteroidal anti-inflammatories; speeds up liver metabolism and breakdown of other medications such as phenytoin and digitoxin

phenylpropanolamine (I) do not use with phenothiazine tranquilizers

phenytoin (I) numerous medications lower the blood levels of phenytoin, e.g., antihistamines, phenobarbital, and antacids; conversely blood levels are increased by the action of phenylbutazone, cimetidine, aspirin products, glucocorticoids, and sulfonamide antibacterials; concurrent use with primidone increases chances of liver toxicity

phosphate enemas (C) extreme care should be taken when used in dogs with serious kidney disease

piperazine (C) do not use in dogs with severe liver or kidney disorders

pilocarpine (C) do not use in dogs with glaucoma or severe heart disease

potassium bromide (C) do not use in dogs with severe renal disease

potassium bromide (I) do not use with spironolactone

potassium citrate (C) same as potassium bromide

potassium citrate (I) same as potassium bromide

primidone (C) care should be taken when used in dogs with a history of liver disease

primidone (I) concurrent use with phenytoin increases chances of liver toxicity; the effectiveness of primidone is increased when used concurrently with antihistamines or chloramphenicol; allergy patients may need higher levels of glucocorticoids if placed on primidone

procainamide (I) should not be used simultaneously with digoxin

prochlorperazine (C) do not use in dogs with enlarged prostates or glaucoma

prochlorperazine (I) do not use in dogs being treated with quinidine

propranolol (C) propranolol is used to treat heart arrhythmias but should not be used in diabetic dogs, or those dogs that are in congestive heart failure

propranolol (I) dogs being treated with propranolol may experience excessive and dangerous low blood pressures if concurrently medicated with furosemide, cimetidine, or phenotiazine products

pyrantel pamoate (C) do not use in dogs with severe liver disease

pyrantel pamoate (I) do not use simultaneously with piperazine as their actions are antagonistic

quinidine (C) care should be used when used in dogs with a history of liver disease

quinidine (I) should not be used with phenithiszine products; care should be taken when used concurrently with digoxin as this product increases the effectiveness of digoxin; phenytoin and phenobarbital decrease the effectiveness of quinidine

spironolactone (C) do not use in dogs with severe renal disease

spironolactone (I) spironolactone increases the effectiveness of digoxin and its dosage may therefore need to be lowered; spironolactone is a diuretic and speeds up the excretion of many products that are eliminated through the kidneys; when used concurrently, aspirin products decrease its effectiveness

stanozolol (C) do not use in pregnant bitches; extreme care should be taken when used in dogs with a history of kidney, liver, or heart disease; do not use in dogs with potentially malignant forms of cancer

stanozolol (I) when used in diabetics, insulin dosage may decrease

sulfonamide antibacterials (I) sulfa-containing products should be used with care in dogs with a history of impaired kidney function; do not use in dogs with "dry eye syndrome" (i.e., keratitis sicca); do not use potentiated forms (i.e., when sulfas are combined with trimethoprim or ormetoprim) in hypothyroid dogs

sulfonamide antibacterials (I) concurrent use with urinary acidifiers or phenothiazines potentially increases the possibility of toxic effects occurring within the kidneys; concurrent use of oral antacids decreases absorption of sulfas by the gastrointestinal tract

tetracycline antibiotics (C) do not use in pregnant bitches or in young dogs during times when their teeth and bones are developing; should not be used in dogs with severe kidney disease

tetracycline antibiotics (I) the absorption of tetracyclines by the gastrointestinal tract is decreased if they are given concurrently with foods or other products high in calcium and antacids; do not use with penicillin, cephalosporin, or aminoglycoside antibiotics as their actions are antagonistic; tetracyclines slow down the liver's metabolism of many products that are broken down or altered by that organ and therefore may alter their dosage; in diabetics tetracycline usage may lower the dosage of insulin

thiabendazole (I) inhibits the metabolism of aminophylline in liver, therefore lowering the dosage needed

timolol maleate (C) do not use in pregnant or lactating bitches; do not use in dogs with a history of severe liver or kidney disease

tylosin (I) concurrent use may decrease digitalis dosage levels

viokase (I) concurrent use of antacids decreases effectiveness

References

Allen, Dana G., John K. Pringle, Dale Smith, and Peter D. Conlon. *Handbook of Veterinary Drugs*. Philadelphia: J. B. Lippincott Company, 1993.

Arthur, Geoffrey H., David E. Noakes, and Harold Pearson. *Veterinary Reproduction and Obstetrics*. 6th ed. London: Bailliere Tindall, 1983.

Barragry, Thomas B. *Veterinary Drug Therapy*. Malvern, Pa.: Lea & Febiger, 1994.

Bistner, Stephen I., and Richard B. Ford. *Kirk and Bistner's Handbook of Veterinary Procedures & Emergency Treatment*. 6th ed. Philadelphia: W. B. Saunders Company, 1995.

Bonagura, John D., editor. *Kirk's Current Veterinary Therapy XII Small Animal Practice*. Philadelphia: W. B. Saunders, 1995.

Booth, Nicholas H., and Leslie E. McDonald, editors. *Veterinary Pharmacology and Therapeutics*. 6th ed. Ames, Ia.: Iowa State University Press, 1988.

Ettinger, Stephen J., and Edward C. Feldman. *Textbook of Veterinary Internal Medicine*, vols. I, II. 4th ed. Philadelphia: W. B. Saunders Company, 1995.

Gelatt, Kirk N. *Veterinary Ophthalmology*. 2nd ed. Malvern, Pa.: Lea & Febiger, 1991.

Georgi, Jay R., and Marion E. Georgi. *Canine Clinical Parasitology*. Malvern, Pa.: Lea & Febiger, 1991.

Greene, Craig E. *Infectious Diseases of the Dog and Cat*. Philadelphia: W. B. Saunders Company, 1990.

Kirk, Robert W., editor. *Current Veterinary Therapy IX Small Animal Practice*. Philadelphia: W. B. Saunders Company, 1986.

Lorenz, Michael D., and Larry M. Cornelius. *Small Animal Medical Diagnosis*. 2nd ed. Philadelphia: J. B. Lippincott Company, 1993.

243

Lorenz, Michael D., Larry M. Cornelius, and Duncan C. Ferguson. *Small Animal Medical Therapeutics.* Philadelphia: J. B. Lippincott Company, 1992.

The Merck Veterinary Manual. 7th ed. Rahway, N.J.: Merck & Company, 1991.

Morgan, Rhea V., editor. *Handbook of Small Animal Practice.* 2nd ed. Philadelphia: W. B. Saunders Company, 1992.

Morrow, David A. *Current Therapy in Theriogenology 2: Diagnosis, Treatment, and Prevention of Reproductive Diseases in Small and Large Animals.* Philadelphia: W. B. Saunders Company, 1986.

Physician's Desk Reference. 49th ed. Montvale, N.J.: Medical Economics Data Production Company, 1995.

Prescott, John F., and J. Desmond Baggot, editors. *Antimicrobial Therapy in Veterinary Medicine.* 2nd ed. Ames, Ia.: Iowa State University Press, 1993.

Scott, Danny W., William H. Miller, Jr., and Craig E. Griffin. *Muller & Kirk's Small Animal Dermatology.* 5th ed. Philadelphia: W. B. Saunders Company, 1995.

Sloss, Margaret W. *Veterinary Clinical Parasitology.* 4th ed. Ames, Ia.: Iowa State University Press, 1970.

Veterinary Pharmaceuticals and Biologicals. 8th ed. Lenexa, Kans: Veterinary Medicine Publishing Company, 1993.

Index

Brand names are set in *italics*.